DR. RADER'S NO-DIET PROGRAM FOR PERMANENT WEIGHT LOSS

William Rader
M.D.

DR. RADER'S NO-DIET PROGRAM FOR PERMANENT WEIGHT LOSS

Published by J. P. TARCHER, Inc.
Los Angeles
Distributed by HOUGHTON MIFFLIN Co.
Boston

Library of Congress Cataloging in Publication Data

Rader, William, 1938–
Dr. Rader's no-diet program for permanent weight loss.

Bibliography: p. 233
Includes index.
1. Reducing—Psychological aspects.
2. Behavior modification. I. Title.
RM222.2.R320 613.2'5'019 79–66688
ISBN 0–87477–139–0

Library of Congress Catalog Card No.: 79-66688

Design by Barbara Monahan

Manufactured in the United States of America

Published by J. P. Tarcher, Inc.
9110 Sunset Blvd., Los Angeles, Calif. 90069

s 10 9 8 7 6 5 4 3 2

No man or woman
feels as worthwhile
as he or she truly is.

Contents

Acknowledgments

I wish to thank July Hollis, a friend, fellow therapist, and recovering compulsive overeater, whose spirit, inspiration, and information were greatly responsible for my evolvement in the field of compulsive overeating. I also want to thank the many patients and the dedicated staff I have worked with in both alcoholism and compulsive overeating programs, as well as the members of Overeaters Anonymous and Alcoholics Anonymous who have been generous with their insights and experiences. Finally, I am grateful for the collaboration of Richard Trubo, who made important editorial contributions in the preparation of this book.

PART 1

THE PRINCIPLES BEHIND THE PROGRAM

1

Permanent Weight Loss Without Dieting

In a culture that worships thinness, constantly bombarding us with media images of slender men and women with adolescent body shapes, it is not surprising that millions of people have turned the weight-loss business into a multi*billion*-dollar industry. At any particular time, there are at least 200 diet books in print. Grocery stores are crammed with sugar-free drinks and low-calorie frozen dinners. Sporting-goods shops are filled with exercise machines. There is an endless number of health spas and "fat farms" aimed exclusively at the overweight.

But even though our society glorifies lean bodies, everywhere we turn there is something to trigger our salivary glands—from the food commercials on TV, to the candy machines in the lunchroom at work, to the sight of McDonald's Golden Arches. It came as no surprise, then, when the U.S. Public Health Service recently reported that some 40 to 80 million Americans are presently obese, making excess weight "one of the most prevalent health problems in the United States today."

A recent *Glamour* magazine survey revealed that 95 percent of its female readership are dieting (mostly unsuccessfully) at least part of the time. Yet only 6 percent of the chronic dieters among us manage to keep their lost pounds off permanently. Even though we claim to be a nation of runners, tennis players, and calorie counters, permanent weight control has been as inaccessible to most people as a distant galaxy. The current state of the art of weight reduction is flawed and failing.

Look at your own "track record" with the conventional approaches. As you've eventually regained even more weight with each new diet you've tried, you have felt upset and defeated. My experience with chronic dieters has shown that this negative reinforcement—the constant reminder of your inability to succeed—can affect your self-confidence and self-esteem, making it even more difficult for you to take control of your life and lose weight for good.

It's time you tried something totally different. I want you to throw away the crash diets and find yourself a friend—a partner—who is as determined to lose weight as you are. Together, you will explore and resolve the many factors that may be contributing to your overweight. The No-Diet Program for Permanent Weight Loss has been successful for hundreds of people. Give yourself a chance to join them.

Sharon, a career woman in her mid-30s, had never been more than fifteen pounds overweight, but she was obsessed with dieting. Every couple of months, she went on a new "quick-weight-loss" diet. From her years of unsuccessful dieting schemes, she had memorized all the facts about nutrition and weight loss: which foods had how many calories, what to eat and what to avoid, how many calories she could consume a day to lose weight, and what constituted a "sensible" portion of food. But within a week of starting each new diet, she would break the regimen, eating long past the point of satiation. And each time she overate, she felt guilty about her "lack of willpower" and depressed about the way she looked, making her eat even more to try to suppress her unhappiness. Sharon was eating compulsively—out of control and against her will.

During the late-night hours, Andrew was totally helpless around food. Through most of the day, he was so busy at the office that he rarely had time to overeat. But about midnight, when the rest of the family was tucked into bed, he would raid the refrigerator and the pantry, eating leftovers, sandwiches, sweets—anything he could find. "My family and friends couldn't understand it," said Andrew. "They never saw me overeat. It all happened at night when no one else was around. The urge was so uncontrollable that it was almost unconscious. I felt like a zombie. I didn't want to do it, but night after night I couldn't stop." Andrew, too, was a compulsive overeater.

For much of their lives, these people had futilely battled the problem of excess weight. Several times a year, each would lose a few pounds on one of the more popular fad diets—the Yogurt Diet, the Grapefruit Diet, the Liquid Protein Diet, the No-Breakfast Diet—only to slip back into their overeating patterns. Without exception, they would gain back all the weight they had lost—and more. Their eating habits, both admitted, were out of control, and each excess pound intensified their unhappiness.

But Sharon and Andrew are now among the hundreds of overweight men and women who have not only lost the extra weight that had burdened them for years, but have also learned to maintain that weight loss *permanently.* Their success can be credited not to a diet, but rather to a multifaceted approach to weight control that is different from any other you've probably experienced—a unique no-diet, partnership approach based on my observation that most chronic dieters suffer from a disorder named the *polymorph syndrome*.

THE POLYMORPH SYNDROME

The plight of most overweight people is strikingly similar, whether they have ten or a hundred pounds to lose. They have generally tried countless diets in the past, some of which helped them lose weight. But regardless of the diet they chose, they have never been able to keep the weight off. Consequently, their weight continually fluctuates up and down—week by week, month by month, year after year. And each time they regain the pounds they've lost, they add on a few more.

To describe this phenomenon, I use the term "polymorph syndrome" (*poly* = many; *morph* = size) to describe the group of symptoms characteristic of the chronic dieter—that is, the fluctuating weight and shape of the person who has struggled unsuccessfully with diet schemes much of his or her life.

The polymorph syndrome has a number of clear psychological and physiological components, which will be described fully in the next two chapters of this book. But its most important—and possibly most distressing—aspect is its compulsive nature. This is the focus of the No-Diet Program and a universal characteristic of the polymorph.

Most overweight people are compulsive overeaters—that is, they are compelled to eat by a strong, irresistible impulse that often runs counter to their conscious will and desire. They eat excessively, often inexplicably and irrationally—eating when they're full, eating "forbidden foods" (sweets, starches, etc.), bingeing in private. Compulsive overeaters have literally lost control over their consumption of food. And they can no more regain conscious control than a diabetic can consciously control his blood-sugar level or a victim of cardiovascular disease can consciously repress a heart attack.

The most common symptoms of polymorphism are listed below. If you are a chronic dieter, you'll probably be able to identify with most of them.

1. Have you made repeated efforts to lose weight, only to eventually regain even *more* pounds than you lost?
2. Do you sometimes eat compulsively in private?

3. Do you eat when you're not hungry, simply because it's "mealtime"?
4. Do you often go on eating binges?
5. Do you feel guilty when you eat too much?
6. Are you often preoccupied with thoughts of food, eating, dieting, or your body shape?
7. Do you eat to comfort yourself from the stresses, anxieties, or troubles in your life?
8. Do you seem to gain weight more easily than other people do, and have more trouble losing it?
9. Have your excess weight or eating habits changed or interfered with the way you live your life?
10. Do you tell yourself that you certainly could lose weight, if you only put your mind to it?

If your responses to at least half of these questions were positive, you—like millions of other people—are suffering from the polymorph syndrome. You are eating compulsively and feel that your lack of willpower is to blame for your excess pounds. But that's not the case. From my experience with patients, it is clear that polymorphs have really lost their power of choice over food. Just like the alcoholic who has a drink or the gambler who plays the horses despite his best intentions not to, you have little control over your own eating behavior. Although you have made endless promises to yourself "never to overeat again," you *can't* eat just a small portion of food when more is available, a single scoop of ice cream when there's a quart in the freezer.

This problem can ultimately be controlled, but it must first be recognized and properly identified. And that means accepting some concepts that may seem foreign to you today. For example, after years of treating polymorphs, I have concluded that compulsive overeaters are, by clinical definition, suffering from a disease, a physical and psychological disorder that is beyond their conscious control. *Disease* is an intimidating word, I know, but it merely describes a condition in which certain bodily processes are functioning improperly. And by *over*eating, you are demonstrating that some physiological or psychological systems are not operating efficiently. This malfunction can include many things, from "overriding" the appetite-regulating mechanism in the brain, to the body's unhealthy dependence on sweet foods, to an uncontrollable need to eat for psychological reasons.

This book, then, focuses not only on the psychological aspects of overeating, but also deals with the physiological components of "polymorphism." For example, if you are overweight, you probably have three to five times as many "fat cells," or adipose tissue, as your thin friends do. This condition has existed since childhood, making it easier for you to gain weight and harder for you to lose it. You are probably also addicted to sugar—a literal physiological and psychological dependency that gives you addictive cravings and withdrawal symptoms when sugar consumption is curtailed. You may even be compelled to overeat by your body's overproduction of a natural substance called "endorphin," which in animal studies has been found in high levels in the brain matter of overweight subjects.

As you proceed through this book, you will come to better understand the many elements that constitute the polymorph syndrome. And when you do, it will become easier for you to acknowledge and accept that your overweight is more than self-indulgence or a lazy will; it is a compulsive disease, like alcoholism, which is unquestionably subject to control. Even so, some people complain that the disease label makes their problem sound graver than they think it really is. "I just figured that I needed to cut down the size of my meals and lose a few pounds," an overweight businessman told me. "But when you introduced the disease concept, it made me feel very uncomfortable. I had thought I just had a character defect. Anyone should be able to lick thirty pounds of weight." Another patient reacted angrily at first: "I didn't want it to be anything as serious-sounding as a disease. But at the same time, I guess it was also reassuring to know *I* wasn't to blame."

For years, you have probably criticized yourself because of your excess weight. And your self-esteem has suffered. But no one tells you that you're weak-willed or lazy if you have arthritis or some other "accepted" disease. And even alcoholism has finally been acknowledged as a disease, and not simply a lack of willpower, by the American Medical Association. Unfortunately, very few doctors recognize yet that overweight is a disease of epidemic proportion in this country, and until they finally do, millions of people will continue to suffer the unhappiness, disappointment, and lack of self-respect that so often are part of the polymorph syndrome.

"Once I realized that my eating behavior was out of my control, it took the shame and guilt out of it," one woman told me. Your entire attitude changes when you can say, "It's not my fault that I'm overweight. It's no one's fault. But it is my responsibility to do something about it." Recognizing this fact will relieve you of an enormous emotional burden that you may have carried around for years, a burden so anxiety-producing that it actually may have kept you overeating.

WHY A NO-DIET PROGRAM?

My clinical experience with overweight patients has convinced me that the only way to permanently lose your extra pounds is to learn to live more normally with food. The No-Diet Program for Permanent Weight Loss is a successful approach to achieve this goal. I'm far from impressed by the results of gimmicky diets with catchy names, like the Calories-Don't-Count Diet, the Drinking Man's Diet, the Quick-Energy Diet, the Liquid Protein Diet, the Grapefruit Diet, or the Zen Macrobiotic

Diet. Nor do I believe in therapeutic modalities like the appetite-suppressant drugs prescribed by most so-called diet experts. Millions of overweight people have tried these popular approaches again and again, and they have universally found that *none of them ever works permanently.* When you "go on" a diet or a drug regimen. it is something that you must eventually "come off." At that point, the weight inevitably returns, too. No diet or pill provides a long-term solution to overweight.

That is why this is not a diet book. Instead, it is a ten-week program that will help people change their patterns of eating for good. This no-diet program will help you and a partner explore the reasons *why* you eat—the psychological causes of your overeating. I will also teach you to understand and short-circuit the connection between your psychological state and food intake, and it will help you learn to live intelligently with food. No special diets, no drugs. Just ten weeks of learning about the polymorph's unique relationship to food.

You will proceed through this plan with a friend whom you'll meet with twice a week and speak to daily by telephone for ongoing insight, support, friendship, and encouragement. You'll talk with this friend about the potent forces that have played a role in your own weight gains. You'll exercise and relax together, and you'll develop your own sensible lifetime eating plans—the antithesis of the crash diets that you've probably tried unsuccessfully dozens of times. In the process, you will lose the weight that you have struggled against for years; and, as your eating habits change, your excess pounds will drop off—and stay off.

It may surprise you to learn that *you really don't need a diet to lose weight permanently.* Your new eating habits must only reflect moderation, not martyrdom. The medical evidence is overwhelming that you can sustain neither weight loss nor good health with a diet that deprives your body of essential nutrients; starves you of a balance of life-supporting carbohydrates, protein, fats, and vitamins; or places you on a regimen of potentially harmful drugs. At worst, you can suffer severe side effects as a result of these weight-loss schemes. At best, you'll lose interest or decide to "reward" yourself with a rich meal—and gain all the weight right back. Learning to eat normally is the only way that your eating habits, and thus your weight loss, will ever become permanent.

In this program, then, you will not be counting calories. Instead, you will be developing a new self-awareness. You are probably not even conscious of your present eating patterns and the self-defeating habits you have developed. One of your partner's roles is to help you recognize this negative eating behavior, as a first step toward changing it. Both of you will discuss the psychological history of your overeating, when and where you eat, what triggers your eating, and how to alter these patterns. Together, you can recondition and reprogram yourselves to eat more healthfully and lose weight in the process.

At the end of this ten-week program, your new eating habits will become as automatic as your inappropriate eating is now. In time, changes in your body's physiology will result in a lessened desire for food. But, more important, with the help of the program you will come to terms with the psychology of your overeating, divest yourself of your negative food habits, and learn a more controlled relationship to food. There will also be an important side benefit: new insights you gain about yourself through the no-diet program will allow your life to be fuller and richer in *all* areas.

YOUR NO-DIETING PARTNER

In this program, you will need to put aside much of what you have previously heard, read, and taken as fact about obesity and weight loss. As a physician and a psychiatrist, I've never accepted the idea that there are magical solutions to chronic problems like overweight. Instead, in this book, you'll find a concrete, ten-week No-Diet program that will teach you, step by step, to help overcome and control the complex physical and psychological barriers that have obstructed your weight loss for so long.

The foundation of this program, once again, is the "partnership system." You will find a fellow polymorph, a friend (I don't recommend relatives, for reasons I'll discuss later) who is also a compulsive overeater, and move through the program together. Or even better, you will join with several partners, and implement the ten-week plan as a group.

Many people are concerned about the partnership aspect of this plan. "I'm embarrassed at the thought of talking about my overweight problem with someone else," they say, or "Can't I do it myself?" Doing it "on your own" has never worked for you in the past—as hard as you've tried and as dedicated as you've always been at the start.

As you will recognize clearly in the weeks ahead, a partner is essential to guide you toward becoming aware of and overcoming the network of factors that have contributed to your chronic overweight condition, the polymorph syndrome. You will discuss with each other areas that may rarely reach your conscious awareness and bring to light other subjects that, by yourself, you might try to avoid. For instance, how do you really feel about being overweight? How would you describe your self-image, and how has it changed since you became overweight? How do you regard your family, parents, friends, and co-workers, and has your relationship with them caused you anxiety or frustration that may provoke overeating behavior?

As you discuss such subjects with your partner, you will rely on each other for insight, strength, encouragement, and empathy. And you'll discover that no one—not even a physician—understands your disorder better than another polymorph. These shared insights will reassure you while helping you change your behavior and learn to control your polymorphism.

This ten-week program can work for you if you are willing to give it a chance. Two partners, Denise and Michelle, lost thirty-seven pounds and eighteen pounds, respectively, with each other's help. They had both tried many diets in the past, without any long-lasting success. They were skeptical—and a bit embarrassed—when they began the program, but that initial apprehension ended quickly.

"The first time we met, when we talked about our overweight problem, I heard my own feelings and my own experiences coming out of Michelle's mouth," recalls Denise. "The pain I felt about being overweight was not mine alone. I didn't feel so isolated. And it made me feel better about myself. Here I was sitting across the table from someone I really thought a lot of—and she was going through the same things I was!"

After a couple of face-to-face meetings, these two women quickly realized they could rely upon one another. "We became each other's twenty-four-hour life-support system," says Denise. "And whenever one of us felt like reaching for some food that wasn't on our eating plan, we could call up the other one and talk about it. My emotional support used to come from food; now it's coming from Michelle."

Most patients tell me that it takes some time to get acquainted with the psychological aspects of their compulsive overeating. After all, they've often never confronted it before, and they're apprehensive about revealing thoughts and feelings to each other which they've even kept hidden from themselves. You and your partner will have to work hard together, particularly in the beginning. But like the jogger whose mile run becomes so much easier after the third week, this program will become more comfortable and rewarding with the passage of time. You'll even find yourself looking forward to your meetings together.

"I thought talking intimately to another person about myself would be the most difficult thing I'd ever done," recalls 40-year-old James, who ultimately and permanently lost fifty-five pounds. "And there was some tension during the first few meetings with my partner. But as we began to see how much we had in common, communicating not only became easy, it became enjoyable. We had each other to lean on, and that made it easier than it had ever been for me to stick to an eating program that would help me lose weight."

In Chapter 4, which explores the partnership system in depth, I will discuss the reasons that this type of peer counseling has been so successful not only with polymorphs, but with many types of physical and psychological disorders. But at this point, let me reassure you that I have personally seen it work not only with overweight people in my own practice and in programs like Overeaters Anonymous, but also while I was chief psychiatrist for the U.S. Navy's alcoholism program and while I was treating kidney-transplant patients. Without question, when peers share a common set of experiences, their understanding, concern, encouragement, and support are the best way of helping one another take responsibility for their overeating and lose weight permanently.

2

The Psychology of Polymorphism

Millie used to begin every day seated before her bathroom mirror applying makeup. Once she stepped away from the mirror, she would get dressed without glancing in it again. At twenty pounds overweight, Millie didn't like the way the rest of her looked. She would wear loose-fitting clothes—long blouses or kaftans—to camouflage the excess weight she detested. "I considered myself a master of disguises—concealing, covering, minimizing my weight," she told me. "I could make my face look pretty, but there wasn't much I could do about the rest of me."

Millie's dilemma was not an isolated phenomenon. Before Cynthia lost her thirty excess pounds, she would dawdle endlessly in front of her closet each morning, trying to choose the most concealing clothes to wear. "I used to wear sweaters on hot days because they hid more," she says. "And I'd wear tent dresses. That way, I could convince myself I really wasn't fat, after all."

Because fatness and thinness manifest themselves most obviously as physical phenomena, it's not surprising that society's focus is upon their physiological components. Most weight-loss books, for example, concentrate exclusively on diets, calories, food groups, and forbidden foods on the assumption that by following a prescribed regimen and using willpower you can lose as much weight as you like. But as you probably know from personal experience, those approaches simply do not work in the long run.

Most weight-loss programs ignore the psychological components of this condition—the effect that overweight has on self-esteem and particularly the compulsive aspect of overeating, which I discussed in the first chapter. If you are a polymorph, you are eating in irrational ways—perhaps going on secret binges or eating when you are no longer hungry. In a very real sense, you have lost the power of choice over food. Your eating behavior is out of your conscious awareness and often beyond your control.

My No-Diet Program for Permanent Weight Loss, however, will gradually teach you how to manage every aspect of your polymorphism. Because peer counseling is the best approach to managing this syndrome, you will use your partner's support to explore—perhaps for the first time—your compulsive eating behavior. You and your partner will help one another recognize facts about your respective relationships with food that you were never aware of before. Only by understanding overeating's causes and effects can you eventually hope to control it, and learn to eat normally and rationally.

In the next few pages, I will discuss the emotional dynamics of the polymorph syndrome that may contribute to your compulsive overeating. You will probably find yourself identifying with much of the discussion in this chapter, and, in the upcoming weeks, you and your partner will discuss many of these same issues as steps toward altering your eating habits.

EATING AS AN EMOTIONAL RESPONSE

Many polymorphs begin eating compulsively in response to emotional turmoil in their lives. For them, the ultimate anxiety-reliever is food. Here is the way the cycle usually works. An individual, troubled by stresses and anxieties in his life, starts eating as a way of coping with his problems. In a real sense, food becomes his tranquilizer, his comforter. But on some level, he knows he shouldn't be overeating and begins to recognize what the excess food is doing to his weight. So he starts feeling guilty, inadequate, and depressed, thus compounding the stress. To escape his growing burdens, he turns again and again to overeating for comfort. When he does, his increasing consumption of food only makes him more depressed and more guilty, further shattering his self-respect as he puts on even more weight. This coping mechanism has obviously created more dilemmas than it has solved.

The self-destructive cycle goes on and on. In the process, the polymorph never faces the real issues—the original life problems that may have initially lured him to overeating. His only escape from this injurious spiral is to resolve those primary issues. As you will find out in this program, if this can be done, the problems of overeating and the excess weight usually resolve themselves as well.

In this program, I will ask you to explore some of the conflicts in your life that may be causing you to overeat. One polymorph discovered that she "binged" every time she returned home from a visit with her mother. Food was her way of coping with the stresses that surfaced during each mother-daughter confrontation. Another polymorph learned that his compulsive overeating occurred primarily when he was studying for exams in college as a means of dealing with the pressures of tests. Still another polymorph, a homemaker, nibbled all day as a result of the frustration and loneliness of being at home by herself.

The mechanism that draws us to eat like this has its roots firmly planted in each of our histories. For example, mothers choose food as the most frequent response to their children's distress. When you cried as an infant, usually you were given a breast or a bottle. That gave you comfort, even if it didn't satisfy whatever may have been your original need.

As you grew older, you were rewarded with candy or a

cookie when you were good. At Christmas, Thanksgiving, birthdays, and other special occasions when you felt very comfortable and loved, food was a major part of the experience as well. On every holiday, your mother would probably cook something everyone really liked, indirectly teaching you to equate, at some level, food with caring. You also grew up with advertisements proclaiming that soups, stews, cakes, cookies, and homemade bread were the best ways to "show your family that you love them."

Throughout your childhood, then, eating became more than just a way to nourish yourself. It was a demonstration of family affection, caring, and security. A full stomach came to mean everything was okay; an empty stomach took on the implication of insecurity and an absence of love. The connection between food and love became a firm part of your experience and your expectations.

No wonder, then, that later in life so many people learn to use food as a substitute for love. A compulsive overeater who is now a therapist working with overweight patients recently told me of the loneliness and isolation she had felt throughout high school and college. She had difficulty making friends and, for many years, food was her closest and most loyal companion. She had gone to college initially to become a dietician so she could always be near food ("I binged all the way through school"). For this woman, eating was clearly a way of giving herself love, which she believed no one else would provide; eventually she learned otherwise, began receiving emotional nourishment from people, and lost all her excess weight.

One of the ironies of the polymorph syndrome is that long after the pleasurable taste of food has waned, the psychological desire for food persists. As I have said repeatedly, overeaters often eat past the point of satiation. Some have told me that even when they feel bloated, nauseated, and disgusted with food, they keep eating. They are eating compulsively, for emotional gratification—the feeling of warmth, security, and comfort that food temporarily provides.

It may be difficult for the nonpolymorph, who has never gotten "drunk on food," to comprehend that anyone could keep eating long after the experience has ceased being pleasant. But a 44-year-old homemaker recalled, "I'd binge on anything sweet. Once I'd start eating, I couldn't stop. I could eat a box of cookies before I'd even realize what I'd done. But even though I'd eat a lot, I didn't taste much. It was almost as though my tastebuds were numb. I don't think I really enjoyed eating that much, and I always felt terrible afterward." To some extent, the ability to avoid reaching for those cookies—whether it be a handful or an entire box—is not within the control of the compulsive over-eater.

Another polymorph, although never more than fifteen pounds overweight, had a similar experience. "When I binged, I was a totally different person," he says. "It was like a rush, like adrenaline flowing through my body. After the first bite, I never even tasted the food. There was never the thought of throwing out food or leaving some for the next day." Even though bingeing has some short-lived psychological value, it is an unproductive and self-destructive way to meet one's emotional needs.

This program is designed to make you conscious of these types of eating behaviors as the first step to abandoning them. A food diary you will keep will make you clearly aware of how you eat in response not just to hunger, but to all types of external stimuli. Early in this ten-week program, many people discover that they have learned to eat in response to certain cues—when watching TV, at social events, whenever they pass an ice cream shop, and at particular times of the day. Under these circumstances, they eat "out of sync" with their physiological requirements, consuming food even when their stomachs are full.

A recent experiment explored this phenomenon, using two groups of people as subjects—overweight persons and those of normal weight. All the subjects were asked to take a general-interest test, which kept them occupied for fifty minutes. At the end of the test, a random sampling in each of the two groups was told it was thirty minutes *later* than it actually was (and thus closer to mealtime), while the others were informed it was thirty minutes *earlier* than real time. Simultaneously, everyone was offered crackers to eat.

The reactions of the overweight people were consistently different from those of the normal-weight group. When obese subjects were told it was close to mealtime, they ate twice as many crackers as the obese people who believed it was earlier than actual time. By contrast, normal-weight individuals from both groups did not exhibit this behavior of eating by the clock, but simply responded to their own personal hunger signals.

If you are a polymorph, this eating pattern may sound familiar to you. The overweight people in the study tended to eat simply because it was "time to eat," not necessarily because they were hungry. Compulsive overeaters have learned to respond not to physiological needs for food, but to external cues like the clock.

The No-Diet Program will help you confront issues like this and teach you how to reverse that conditioning. Unless you are on a thorough program that deals with all aspects of your disorder, you will probably never untangle the learned behaviors and the life stresses that are causing your overeating. And until you do, even if you lose weight on a particular crash diet, you will eventually regain it all and, in your frustration and disappointment, turn to even more food, again using it as a comforter/tranquilizer. Food, for the compulsive overeater and chronic dieter, is a defense against anxiety. And, in clinical terms, until you confront the causes of your overeating you will "move in the direction of the defense" you have relied on for so many years.

This entire scenario, with all its emotional and behavioral components, may sound exaggerated. Perhaps you can't imagine that it really applies to you. But I am sure it does, at least to some degree. Millions of overweight people cope with stress precisely that way. It's true that you do not engage in any of this behavior consciously—that is, you don't make a decision to overeat to soothe yourself after a bad day at the office. However, without recognizing it, that is likely to be exactly what you do.

To demonstrate how compulsive and irrepressible this type of behavior can sometimes become, let me relate the story of one polymorph who, at age 38, on his son's fifth birthday, received a physical examination. He weighed over 300 pounds at the time of that visit. "Unless you lose a lot of weight," his physician warned, "you'll never live to see your son's tenth birthday. Don't make me sign your death certificate." The man was so panicky when he left the doctor's office that he turned to his most reliable friend—food—to comfort him. He stopped at a restaurant for a large meal.

Throughout his life, the only way this man had ever dealt with panic—the only tranquilizer that ever worked for him—was food. He had always eaten for the security, the safety, and the numbness it provided. Fortunately, he eventually turned his life around when a friend approached him with a partnership program for weight control. With his friend, he found caring, comfort, and support, and was subsequently able to lose his excess weight—and keep it off.

As irrational and exaggerated as this patient's behavior may seem to you, keep in mind that the polymorph syndrome is a compulsive disease. As I will emphasize again and again throughout this book, if you're a polymorph, asking you to consciously control your overeating is pointless. You have tried to for years—unsuccessfully. You know you should lose weight but it's literally beyond your control to do so on your own.

Rationally, we all know that food is not the best choice we can make to supply us with comfort, love, companionship, and security. You need not be a psychiatrist to recognize that a dish of ice cream or a candy bar cannot replace the caring and the concern of another human being. As you gradually form an intimate relationship with your partner in this no-diet program, you will understand this concept better.

SELF-ESTEEM AND THE DENIAL SYSTEM

When I recently asked a group of polymorphs to describe their feelings about themselves, their answers were predictable: shame, guilt, insecurity, disgust, depression, frustration, pain. Patient after patient told me that, in this fiercely antifat society, they were ashamed of their bodies. Their self-esteem had been so devastated by being overweight—even when by any clinical estimate they had as few as ten or fifteen excess pounds to lose—that happiness and well-being were foreign to them. They strove for perfection—to be number 1—even though such goals are impossible for anyone to attain. They weren't satisfied to be themselves and had internalized the biases, prejudices, and judgments of society, creating their own self-depreciation system. I have seen countless patients who are literally enraged at themselves because they have gained a few pounds or failed on a diet they had staked their hopes on.

Several studies have indicated that this self-esteem problem is particularly intense among overweight women. In our culture, women are still defined and evaluated by their bodies much more than men are. No wonder that rarely does a women's magazine appear without prominently featuring a new diet; in contrast, men's magazines seldom run articles about losing weight.

The female polymorph's displeasure with her body shape often becomes all-consuming and obsessive. She blows her imperfections out of proportion, giving them unfair emphasis when she evaluates herself. Whatever virtues she may possess—intelligence, career success, talent, charm, compassion—are overshadowed by disgust with the way she looks. These negative impressions become her self-image, and she ignores her positive qualities or, at best, relegates them to very secondary importance.

"I can't stay away from the refrigerator," one successful commercial artist in her mid-40s told me, "and I hate myself every time I open the refrigerator door. Sometimes, while I'm eating, I'm cursing myself mentally for the way I look. I feel terrible about what I've done to myself. There's really not much about me that I like anymore."

These kinds of feelings are not really so surprising, whether expressed by men or women. We are all constantly making value judgments about ourselves, consciously or unconsciously. Most often, we make these evaluations by comparing ourselves to others—not only to the people around us, but also to media images of beauty, success, charm, or sexual attractiveness. Magazines, billboards, television, and the movies present us with images of "perfect" men and women—unflawed, unblemished, unbulging. And we accept these unrealistic standards of perfection and feel inadequate and worthless when we don't match up to them.

When a person—polymorph or not—feels bad about himself, it dramatically affects his behavior in the world. He or she unconsciously carries around this crippled self-esteem twenty-four hours a day, influencing efficiency at work, values, goals, mood, relationships, even the ability to love. And in the process, he or she begins feeling depressed, insecure, tense, full of self-doubts.

To cope with their poor self-esteem, and to minimize or avoid the psychological pain that overeating is causing them, polymorphs create their own "denial system." Millie, the woman at the beginning of this chapter who avoided looking at her body, and Cynthia, who dressed in loose-fitting clothes, would not acknowledge the reality of their obesity. Their denial system, like that of other polymorphs, was a defense mechanism to suppress the anxiety and depression that resulted when they recognized that their bodies did not look like they wanted them to. It was a self-protective, coping device to shield themselves from the pain that this problem caused them.

Denying your dilemma may seem less distressing than realistically confronting the poor self-image and psychological problems that may be causing your overeating in the first place. And this denial system can take many forms. You may try to rationalize the problem ("Everyone I know is overweight; it's such a common thing"). Or you may use language that minimizes your overeating ("All I'm going to eat is just a *sliver* of cake and a *dab* of ice cream"). Or you may place the blame for your obesity elsewhere ("My scale has always been way off").

When I explain the connection between lowered self-esteem and the denial system, most polymorphs seem to identify with it immediately and respond with stories of their own. "I had convinced myself that I really wasn't as overweight as I was," explained a young woman. "I never looked at myself in full-length mirrors, so I lived by the lies I told myself. Then one day as I was walking past a store window, I saw the reflection of a very overweight woman in the glass. I remember thinking, 'Oh, that poor fat lady!' A second later, I realized it was me I was looking at. I was horrified!"

Take a moment to evaluate the denial system that you have created for yourself in order to avoid confronting your self-image and your excess weight. Most people tell themselves "white lies" or rationalizations to spare themselves from their reality. They tend to overreact when anyone else refers to a sensitive subject like overweight. Consider whether you sometimes become defensive about your excess pounds. Do you become angry when someone mentions your weight or suggests that you lay off the croissants? Do you try to deceive yourself and others by minimizing your problem? Look over the following statements and see how many you can identify with.

"Sure, I'm bingeing tonight, but I'll fast tomorrow."

"I keep cookies in the house only for the children."

"Everyone gains weight on a vacation."

"I'm not fat; there's just more of me to love."

"I could lose this weight if I really put my mind to it."

"The dryer shrinks all my clothes."

"I didn't have lunch today, so it's okay if I eat a lot tonight."

"I can take another helping of pasta because I turned down the garlic bread."

"It may look like a big portion, but Chinese food is mostly vegetables."

"Bodies were meant to be soft and round."

"I'd rather be fat and happy than thin and miserable."

"It's ridiculous to try looking like a 17-year-old when you're 35."

"I don't need to lose weight; I just need some exercise to tone up my muscles."

If your intention is to lose weight permanently, you must stop this kind of rationalizing, denying, and deceiving. Perhaps for years you and your partner have not perceived yourselves as you really are—not only refusing to acknowledge excess pounds and problem areas in your self-esteem, but also failing to recognize all the positive qualities in your lives. In this ten-week program, you will start seeing yourself in a different light, in a fairer, more balanced way; and, as you do, your self-esteem will gradually improve. You will begin to take responsibility for changing those things you aren't content with, and in the process you will finally lose weight and come to recognize your personal worth.

POLYMORPHISM AND YOUR BEHAVIOR

As you can see, the polymorph syndrome has a complex framework of causes and effects. Not only does the polymorph eat for reasons beyond his conscious awareness, he also *uses* his obesity in a variety of subconscious ways, some of which you will learn about and may identify with in the upcoming weeks of the program.

For instance, I recall a 28-year-old woman named Julaine who insisted that she was quite content with her twenty-five-pound overweight problem, which had persisted for years. True, she periodically went through the motions of going on a diet, but never really made a serious commitment to losing weight. In individual therapy, however, Julaine discovered that she was really not as content as she had told herself she was. She recognized that she had been using her obesity as a defense against sexuality. "I was raised in an old-fashioned way, and grew up with a lot of taboos surrounding sex," she said later. "I got to the point where I was afraid to be sexual. As long as I remained fat, I thought that I had nothing to worry about. No one wants to flirt with a fat lady."

Many psychiatrists and psychologists have recognized that a considerable number of overweight men and women like Julaine are battling unresolved conflicts about their sexuality. Maintaining their excess weight is one means of protecting themselves against sexual activity. Even polymorphs who are very interested in having a satisfying sex life are often unable to find fulfillment. They tend to feel such shame and embarrassment about their weight that they are extremely self-conscious and often dislike being naked, even in front of their mates. When making love, they concentrate primarily on "posing" for their lover, lying just the right way in bed to minimize their bulges. Their concern with how they look sabotages the pleasure they might otherwise find in the sexual experience.

Similarly, when sex is absent or unfulfilling in your life,

food can often become a symbolic substitute for the sexual experience. Eating is a means of putting something stimulating and pleasurable into your body. Therefore, in a sense, food can supply sexual, loving gratification, although obviously not of a true or permanent nature.

In contrast, some polymorphs relate to their sexuality quite differently than Julaine. Rather than using their obesity to protect themselves against male-female encounters, they overindulge in sex to prove to themselves that they are attractive. By being sexually active, they are attempting to counteract their negative self-image, which has usually incorporated many of society's unfair stereotypes about obese people. But because this sexual promiscuity is rarely accompanied by love and intimacy, it leaves the polymorph feeling unfulfilled and frustrated.

In time, many overweight people find themselves becoming isolated. In therapy, a few of my patients have realized that their layer of fat is both a symbolic and an actual means of separating themselves from their environment, and particularly from other people. In extreme cases, they actually prefer complete societal detachment and spend most of their time alone. One man so abhorred competition and had so great a fear of failure that he used his polymorphism to avoid all risk taking. He resigned himself to a job that didn't fulfill his potential but that provided a safe and secure environment. He also stayed away from all social functions because of his obesity, thus avoiding any chance of social failure. He had built a wall between himself and his surroundings.

Polymorphs like this usually view the world as hostile and their large bodies as a fortress against it. They tend to lead solitary lives so that their feelings will rarely be tested and they can maintain an emotional distance from others.

True, this particular phenomenon occurs primarily with the grossly overweight. But even polymorphs who have less dramatic problems may allow their excess weight to influence their choice of friends, subconsciously choosing to associate primarily with people who won't confront or criticize their weight problem. Often, without consciously realizing why, obese people may eliminate thin friends from their social life because they feel threatened or self-conscious in their company. They may rationalize this behavior by explaining that they've allowed certain friendships to die because "I don't like their parties; all they talk about anymore is boring politics" or "They're obsessed with people's bodies—how shallow can you be?" But, in fact, their embarrassment and anxiety over how they look and how others react to it have caused them to dramatically rearrange their interpersonal relationships.

Even as polymorphs adapt to their overweight condition by restructuring their social environment, many never give up the dream that their weight, their relationships—and their life—will eventually become ideal. One woman fantasized, "Someday, when I lose this weight, I'm going to really get involved with life and be successful." Another said, "After I slim down, everything will be just fine. I'll finally get the man I want." Polymorphs often avoid reality by dreaming about tomorrow, all the while fearing that their dreams may never be actualized.

This book offers you a realistic chance to bring your compulsive overeating under control. Although you may have found some of the issues discussed in this chapter complex and possibly even intimidating, with a partner you can find out which areas apply to you and how best to understand and resolve them. With each passing day, focus as much as possible on the "here and now"—concentrating on what is happening that day rather than on past disappointments or future anxieties.

Please be aware that even though the polymorph syndrome has many psychological components, there is no indication that most compulsive overeaters need traditional psychotherapy. You are not mentally ill; you don't need to "have your head examined." Rather, by reading this book and starting the No-Diet Program, you will have exhibited one of the *healthiest* signs you possibly could—a willingness to change, to commit your energies to a permanent revision of your attitudes and the control of your weight.

A partnership approach—finding a friend and moving through this program with him—will be your key to success in the next ten weeks. The effectiveness of peer counseling for compulsive conditions, including overeating, has been substantiated in dozens of studies in recent years. A partner can clearly make your goal of permanent weight control a reality.

If you are now using food to fill voids in your life, or as one of your primary coping mechanisms, I hope that you will soon begin taking responsibility for altering that lifestyle. It is time you started letting people—in this case, your partner—satisfy some of those needs. Once that happens, your compulsive cravings for food will subside and you will begin losing weight for good.

3

The Physiology of Polymorphism

Marilyn had constantly struggled to lose weight throughout adolescence and into her adult life. She could not remember a time when she had not been heavier than she wished to be, and she was always either on a diet or thinking about starting one.

"The most frustrating thing was being around so many friends who could lose weight easily," she explains. "For me, it was almost impossible to lose even five or ten pounds, and when I finally did, I'd gain them back quicker than I lost them. Dieting was like fighting a war that I always seemed to lose."

Marilyn's predicament—and that of other polymorphs—can be explained. I suggested that she start by looking at her own baby pictures. And she was surprised at what she saw. Not only had she been overweight almost from birth, but her obesity had worsened as she grew older. She had *always* weighed more than she should have, and that established a physiological basis that has made it extremely difficult for her to lose weight in adult life.

To complicate the weight-loss aims of polymorphs like Marilyn, many physiological obstacles stand in their way, in addition to the psychological aspects of this disease we have already discussed. Polymorphs must deal with much more than the compulsive behavior, the role that poor self-esteem plays in their overeating, the complex denial system and rationalizations, and the ways that food is used as a substitute for love, comfort, and sexual fulfillment. For example, the number and composition of the polymorph's fat cells make it more difficult to lose weight. Recent theories indicate that an addiction to sugar makes the body crave that high-caloric substance. And a bodily chemical called endorphin may occur in excessive amounts in the polymorph, organically urging him to overeat.

With phenomena like these at work, it is hardly startling that overweight people so often remain obese. The polymorph syndrome is simply too complex to manage alone. This program, fortunately, offers you the tools to succeed and provides a concrete plan to start you eating sensibly.

WHEN ARE YOU OVERWEIGHT?

Most people do not require charts or even scales to tell them they are overweight. All they need do is look at themselves in a full-length mirror or try on last year's wardrobe. These subjective impressions are all that is necessary to convince them that they must lose a few pounds.

The medical profession, however, has devised more scientific methods of determining obesity or, as many physicians call it, "excessive fat deposition." Some of these techniques measure body density (weight per unit of volume); others gauge body water content. Clinical writings tend to define obesity as 20 percent or more over "normal" body weight. But all of these "objective" determinations leave little room for individual variation.

Probably the simplest test—and one that you can do without height-weight charts or a subjective judgment of whether you have a small, medium, or large frame—is the "pinch test." To measure the amount of fat on your own body, locate a spot over your lowest rib, straight down from the armpit. At this point, take a deep pinch of skin between your thumb and index finger. If the fold is more than one inch thick, it is an indication of excessive bodily fat.

I believe that beyond knowing that you are, in fact, overweight, the precise number of excess pounds you have—whether it be fifteen or fifty—is a secondary issue in treating this disorder. No matter how much weight you have to lose, the No-Diet Program will remain unchanged, because it is aimed at helping you understand and resolve the compulsive aspects of your eating habits. The struggle within you is the same whether your weight problem is slight or severe. It should relieve you somewhat, however, to learn the physiology behind why you gain weight so easily and why it's so hard to lose it.

THE FAT-CELL PHENOMENON

Perhaps no physiological factor is more critical to your understanding of the polymorph syndrome than the fat-cell phenomenon. First, let me provide you with some background. For decades, physicians have observed that obesity often "runs in families." According to one study, about 40 percent of children who have one overweight parent are obese themselves; an incredible 80 percent are overweight if *both* their parents are obese. Many doctors concluded, then, that a genetic link accounted for most obesity. It was, they believed, an inherited disorder.

However, another phenomenon gradually became obvious: even when both parents were thin, overweight babies tended to become overweight children and, in turn, overweight adults. In these cases, the weight of the parents appeared irrelevant; much more influential were the child's eating habits. The key here was the number and size of the body's fat cells—adipose tissue—which are largely determined by childhood eating patterns.

Here is what typically happens. As you eat, the food you consume is broken down for use as energy, and any excess calories not used as energy are converted to fat and stored in the body's fat cells. Studies at the Mt. Sinai Medical Center in New York have identified three critical periods of life when fat cells are formed: the three final months in utero; the first two years after birth; and early adolescence. Thus, the more you were fed during childhood, the greater the number of fat cells that were produced by your body. Once these excess cells are formed, they remain a part of you for life, always in want of filling.

If you are a polymorph who overate as a teenager, you may have two to four times as many fat cells as someone who ate moderately during adolescence. While an adult with normal weight may have from 30 to 40 billion fat cells in his body, the polymorph may have from 60 to 160 billion. To compound his difficulties, the polymorph must contend not only with *more* fat cells, but also with the greater fat-storage capacity of each individual cell.

So what happens when the polymorph diets? His weight loss will reduce the size of each existing cell as its fat content is depleted, but the number of cells will remain unchanged. As soon as his diet ends, he will probably begin consuming more food than his body needs for its daily functions. The excess calories will be converted to fat, quickly filling out these permanent receptacles once more.

No wonder Marilyn sometimes complained, "I eat the same amount of food as my friends—why do I gain weight and they don't? I could eat air or feathers and get fat!" Marilyn's fat-cell makeup is probably different from that of her friends. Because she most likely has so many more fat cells, she can eat the *same* amount of food as they do and gain weight.

The fat-cell phenomenon, which is now a universally accepted medical principle, raises some interesting questions, particularly about the child-feeding practices that have endured for generations. We are all familiar with the saying "A fat baby is a healthy baby," but it certainly seems out of date now. Many years ago, a child's weight reserve might have been useful in helping him endure various infectious diseases; today, however, the common childhood illnesses are rarely accompanied by significant weight loss. Even so, most parents still believe that a plump baby is a sign of good health. My firm conviction is that polymorphism would be much less prevalent in the next adult generation if children today grew up eating moderately rather than being overfed.

Finally, new studies have discovered still another phenomenon to help explain why people can eat the same amounts of food, but only some of them will gain weight doing so. Researchers have learned that in certain types of fat cells—called brown fat cells—excess calories are burned off as heat in the normal person, thus maintaining his or her weight at an optimum level. But when this process malfunctions, as in an overweight individual, the excess weight is *not* burned off and is stored as fat. This calorie-burning process is not only less functional in some people than in others, but it also tends to become less effective with age, perhaps explaining the onset of obesity in older people. Scientists are now seeking techniques to promote the proper functioning of brown fat cells.

THE SUGAR-OBSESSED SOCIETY

As if the fat-cell phenomenon were not enough for the compulsive overeater to contend with, research is also beginning to show that polymorphs are addicted to sugar. Addiction, of course, is a word we usually apply to alcoholics, other drug abusers, or chronic cigarette smokers. But some studies now support the theory that sugar can cause a state of addiction just as real as if you were "hooked" on alcohol, heroin, or tobacco.

When you consume large amounts of sugar, your body's

level of insulin (a pancreas-produced hormone) and triglycerides (body fat) gradually elevate, triggering a condition called hypoglycemia (low amounts of glucose in the blood). Soon, the classic symptoms of hypoglycemia (and obesity) start surfacing with varying intensity, including both physiological symptoms (fatigue, feelings of weakness, lightheadedness, drugged or bloated sensations, headaches) and psychological ones (depression, anxiety, tension). Most of the symptoms disappear, ironically, when more sugar is consumed. Thus, sugar itself is used to relieve the very problems it has caused, and a vicious, addictive cycle begins. Some researchers have called this addictive phenomenon "carboholism."

By definition, an addiction occurs when a person succumbs to a practice that is not only habit-forming, but causes withdrawal when the habit is given up. This is certainly true with the alcoholic, the heroin addict, the cigarette smoker—and the polymorph. When you significantly reduce your body's consumption of sugar, you may experience some of the same withdrawal symptoms of other kinds of addictions—headaches, dizziness, shakiness, irritability, nervousness. There is a craving, an agitation, an apprehension, a general malaise, and a definite physiological urge to ease the withdrawal symptoms by eating more sugar-containing substances.

"Sometimes, dieting would actually scare me," recalls Linda, one chronic dieter who followed my program. "I would get depressed and anxious, I had trouble sleeping, and often I had terrible nightmares. There were some physical reactions, too, like shortness of breath, chest pains, cramps. I didn't know what was happening to me. There were times when I'd even quit the diet just because it made me so uncomfortable."

Because of sugar's potentially disruptive impact upon your body and mind, it is unfortunate that the substance is so ubiquitous in the American diet. The average person now consumes 2.4 pounds of sugar per week (as compared to 2.1 pounds of beef) in the foods he eats. Because that is only an average, the polymorph probably consumes even more. And as the polymorph's sugar intake elevates, not only does his weight increase, but so does the severity of the side effects discussed above, as well as the risks of contracting degenerative diseases, from tooth decay to diabetes.

I would like you to contemplate for a moment the many sources of sugar in your own diet. Of course, you're familiar with the obvious—sugar in your coffee, soft drinks, and desserts. But sugar is an ingredient in almost *everything* we eat. The next time you're in the supermarket, try finding packaged food items that *don't* contain sugar. It is an ingredient in breads, salad dressings, lowfat yogurts, fruit juices, applesauce, canned soup, frozen vegetables, breakfast cereals, cottage cheese, chili sauce, ketchup, baby foods, and even salt.

In 1978 alone, food manufacturers used over 12 *billion* pounds of sugar as a food additive. Even if you drink your coffee black and avoid rich desserts, you probably still consume more sugar every day than any other single food substance. And the amounts that are not immediately utilized by your body are converted into fats and stored in your fat cells, causing weight gain.

Sugar consumption, I believe, is not only physiologically addictive, but it is also a conditioned obsession. From childhood, we have *learned* to eat sugar-laden foods. Millions of dollars are spent on TV advertising to encourage children to eat fattening candy bars and sugar-heavy breakfast cereals. Also, as a society, we have designated ice cream and candy as reward foods, symbols of parental love and special accomplishments. By contrast, meat, fish, and fresh fruits and vegetables are usually considered "what you have to eat before you get dessert."

I have never seen any medical evidence that humans physiologically and instinctively prefer sweeter foods over healthier ones. In fact, quite the opposite appears to be true. I am reminded of a study conducted years ago with malnourished children in an orphanage. Bowls of various kinds of food were placed before the children, including both nutritious foods and sweets. The most nutritious foodstuffs were mixed together in a horrible-tasting combination. Even so, the children, given a choice, instinctively selected the bowls that would provide them with balanced nutrition, no matter how bad it tasted. This shows clearly that if there was anything instinctive about their nutritional desires, it was their longing for such essential nutrients as protein, fats, vitamins, and minerals.

Intuitively, and from years of reading about nutrition and dieting, the polymorph knows the best types of food for him, but his instincts and knowledge are overwhelmed by conditioning and a physiological addiction. However, changes in the way you eat *are* possible. As you and your partner become involved in this program, I will ask you both to dramatically reduce the levels of your sugar consumption. Consequently, you can expect to experience some of the withdrawal symptoms that I mentioned earlier. For some polymorphs, withdrawal symptoms are quite severe; for others, they may be barely perceptible. But with your partner's help, you will learn to deal with them and not rush to sugary foods for relief and comfort. Your body will eventually adjust to sugar deprivation, and your cravings for sugar will disappear.

THE APPESTAT AND SATIATION

To thoroughly comprehend why he overeats, the polymorph should be aware of the nerve center within the hypothalamus of the brain called the appestat. When properly functioning, the appestat is a natural, self-regulating means of preventing overeating, for it signals other parts of the brain when the body has consumed all the food it requires. A properly functioning appestat automatically adjusts your appetite to meet your energy needs each day and notifies your body when you have eaten enough. If you repeatedly overeat, however, your appestat is either malfunctioning or is being overpowered by a number of other factors, including the psychological forces that play a role in the polymorph syndrome.

In Gail's childhood, for instance, her mother responded to stress in the young girl's life (whether it was unhappiness, disappointment, anger, or frustration) by giving her food as a tranquilizer. Now, in adulthood, Gail unconsciously reacts by eating whenever she experiences stress, no matter what message her appetite-controlling center may be trying to communicate.

Liza, early in her adult life, developed the habit of eating in the evening while watching television. This behavior became so ingrained in her psyche, and so much a part of her daily routine, that nothing she tried on her own could break this conditioning. The messages from her brain were insignificant in comparison with her compulsive "need" to eat at night as she watched TV.

So even if your appestat is communicating the message of satiation to the brain, you may still overeat, merely because that is how you have unconsciously learned to react to certain life situations.

THE ENDORPHIN CONNECTION

Medicine still has much to learn about compulsive overeating and obesity. And as our knowledge increases, the polymorph syndrome has begun to encompass components that no one ever considered even a decade ago. We now know that the functioning of the appestat is not the only activity in the brain of interest to polymorphs. "Endorphin," for example, is a word that was unheard of until the early 1970s, and yet today there is growing evidence that it may play a major role in obesity.

Endorphins are molecules naturally produced in the brain which, among other properties, have shown signs of turning off pain sensations. But for our purposes, the most interesting phenomenon is that *elevated* levels of endorphins have been found in obese animals. In studies with both rats and mice at Temple University, Tufts University, and the National Institute of Mental Health, twice as much endorphin has been discovered in the pituitaries of overweight laboratory animals as in their thin counterparts. In one study, when endorphins were injected into satiated rats, compulsive eating began within two to five minutes and continued for forty to sixty minutes. After researchers gave these overweight animals an antidote, called naloxone, which neutralized the potency of endorphins, the overeating ceased.

The first human studies investigating the link between obesity and endorphins began in 1980 at the National Institute of Health, and the conclusive findings are still perhaps years away. But the animal research suggests that a relationship between endorphins and overeating may exist. For humans, this indicates still another physiological dimension to the polymorph syndrome. This natural chemical, when produced in excess, may be causing you to overeat.

THE CONVENTIONAL MEDICAL "SOLUTION" TO POLYMORPHISM

If you are like most other polymorphs, after enduring dozens of diets without long-lasting success you have probably arrived at your physician's office at least once, perhaps many times, seeking a solution. However, when most doctors dip into their black bags, they come out with only another diet—or "diet pills." But neither dieting nor appetite suppressants will provide permanent weight control because both methods fail to deal with the compulsive nature of this disorder. Even though the dieter or patient may lose weight temporarily, statistics show that he will regain it once he starts eating "normally" again and resumes his compulsive eating behaviors.

As a polymorph, you are probably familiar with the drugs typically prescribed by physicians in their physiological attack on obesity. The most frequently prescribed diet pills are amphetamines, which account for more than 14 million individual prescriptions a year in this country. Nearly 90 percent of the legal, medical use of amphetamines today is for weight control; they are also prescribed for such disorders as minimal brain dysfunction and a sleep problem called narcolepsy. But the appetite-suppressing properties of amphetamines wane rapidly, and, in the process, various significant side effects can surface—including elevated heart rate and blood pressure, acute anxiety, and even cerebral-vascular disorders leading to brain damage. (I am familiar with several cases of overweight patients who have died of brain hemorrhages caused when blood vessels in the brain weakened and burst, directly attributable to long-term consumption of amphetamines.)

To compound the polymorph's misery, he can even become *addicted* to amphetamines. The majority of these "addicts" are overweight men and women who receive the pills from their physicians. A study by the National Institute on Drug Abuse confirmed that amphetamines are America's most abused prescription drug. The reasons for this are many. To begin with, some physicians are simply not cautious enough when they prescribe drugs like amphetamines. They are not as sensitive as they should be to the physiological dependency that usually occurs with extended use of these pills. Even when doctors eventually suggest that their patients curtail their consumption of the drug, the polymorph experiences such intense withdrawal symptoms—sometimes including severe depression—that he generally begins overeating to pacify himself.

A recent AMA directive on amphetamines and similar drugs said: "Their undesirable effects, including a tendency to produce psychic and, occasionally, physical dependence when used indiscriminately and in large doses, make their use hazardous." If the conservative AMA is so outspoken on the use of "diet pills," the situation is obviously serious. I see no positive aspects to taking these drugs. Appetite suppressants are not the solution for a disease in which hunger is not the problem. As a polymorph, you are overeating for reasons other than biological hunger. In my opinion, you are better off not going to a doctor who approaches weight control with drugs.

Many physicians have admitted to me that they don't know what else to do for overweight people except prescribe pills. True, a carefully controlled drug (but *not* "diet-pill") regimen may be helpful for the few overweight people who have a thyroid hormone deficiency, which disrupts their metabolism, prevents their bodies from properly utilizing food, and leads to increased fatty deposits. For these persons, drugs may stabilize this abnormality. But research at Yale University indicates that this condition is rare—occurring in less than 2 percent of all overweight people—despite the "hormonal" or "thyroid" rationalization frequently used by the polymorph. For the overwhelming majority of the overweight population, most physicians have little to offer.

I am not attempting to indict the medical profession. Doctors have little opportunity to learn about the cause and control of obesity. In medical schools, almost nothing is taught about weight control or nutrition. In their practices, physicians have such limited success helping their overweight patients that most—except for "diet specialists"—are eventually unwilling to spend much time and energy in this ungratifying and frustrating task. And even many of the diet doctors rely almost exclusively on ineffective long-term treatments such as drugs and diets.

Ironically, as the average physician tries unsuccessfully to manage the physiological aspects of polymorphism, still another problem sometimes develops—specifically, the doctor's unconscious sabotage of the very weight-loss program he has prescribed. In the typical physician-polymorph interaction, the doctor, hardly immune from the biases and prejudices of the rest of society, may unconsciously project his personal discomfort for obesity upon his patient. He may be judgmental ("What's wrong? Some of my other patients have lost weight on this diet"). He may blame your problem on a lack of willpower. And he might not offer the encouragement and support that you need. He is not malicious; he wants to help you. He simply does not understand polymorphism and your compulsive eating behavior. And he feels helpless, unable to treat your disorder effectively. He would generally rather care for patients with pneumonia or a broken bone—at least he can heal these ailments.

A patient named Doris related: "One doctor I had, even though he was overweight himself, was very unfair in the way he treated me," she told me. "He spent most of the time talking about my lack of willpower. I had the feeling that he never really saw beyond my layer of fat, and thought of me as only a 'fat person,' not as a person who just happened to be fat. He wasn't understanding at all, and I used to leave his office more depressed than when I went in."

By introducing the concept of polymorphism to the public, and by approaching the management of this disease in a thoroughly different way, it is my hope that the attitude of the medical community will begin to change. Until doctors universally alter their approach to treating the polymorph syndrome, with all of its physiological and psychological components, the disease will continue to persist for millions of people.

POLYMORPHISM'S PHYSIOLOGICAL SIDE EFFECTS

If you are a polymorph, your concern about your excess weight should extend beyond just how you look. As a multidimensional phenomenon, polymorphism can affect your physiological well-being in many ways, no matter how overweight you are. In fact, even if you have only ten or fifteen excess pounds, your body is suffering from the stresses of this overweight and, in the long run, it may be damaged to some degree. For example, there is a much higher death rate from cardiovascular disease—particularly heart attacks—among the overweight because the added burden of too much weight forces the heart to work harder to pump blood through the body. As a polymorph, you may also be experiencing increased cholesterol deposits on the inside walls of your coronary arteries, which can obstruct and eventually block the flow of oxygen to the heart.

Frequent weight loss and gain over short periods of time is actually *more* damaging physically than maintaining a moderate level of excess weight. Studies indicate that, as described above, cholesterol levels in the blood increase during periods of weight gain and fatty deposits are lodged on the walls of essential arteries. But when weight is lost, these deposits do not contract proportionately, and with each subsequent weight gain the blood vessels narrow even further, enhancing the chances of a heart attack. Thus, you are better off remaining moderately overweight than losing and regaining over and over.

Here is the way a U.S. Public Health Service report described this phenomenon: "Repeatedly losing and gaining weight may be more harmful than maintenance of a steady weight at a high level. For example, it has been shown that serum cholesterol levels are elevated during periods of weight gain, thus increasing the risk of deposition [of fatty substances]. We have no evidence to show that once cholesterol has been deposited it can be removed by weight reduction. It is possible that a patient whose weight has fluctuated up and down a number of times has been subjected to more atherogenic stress than a patient with stable though excessive weight. . . . If an animal has once been obese and then has been repeatedly reduced, it will have a shorter life expectancy than an animal which has never been reduced."

The Build and Blood Pressure Study—a long-term study of 5 million individuals concluded in 1959—showed that mortality was one-third higher among men who were 20 percent or more overweight. When the level of excess weight reached 40 percent above average, the risk of mortality jumped to at least 70 percent above normal. Although female mortality was less affected by obesity, overweight women still experienced a noteworthy increase in death rates.

In both sexes, this elevated mortality rate is usually traceable to chronic diseases caused by excess weight. As a polymorph, your chances of developing diabetes, for instance, is significantly greater than if you were normal weight. A thin person may have a prediabetic condition, and yet the disease will never manifest itself because of his proper eating habits; but an overweight person with the same predisposition may become a clinical diabetic simply because of his excessive food intake. Thus, the obese person is running a serious health risk by maintaining his excess weight.

I have treated polymorphs suffering from many other weight-related disorders. When victims of arthritis are overweight, increased strain is placed upon their joints, intensifying pain and reducing mobility. There also appears to be some correlation between cancer and polymorphism, although the evidence is not conclusive. Even so, there is no longer any doubt that managing polymorphism is literally a matter of life and death.

Your body is perpetually seeking an equilibrium, trying to maintain a particular red-blood-cell count, a precise white-cell count, a hormonal balance, an appropriate state of energy use and storage, and so on. Few of us fully realize what an incredibly balanced instrument we are. But when the polymorph's weight fluctuates, these balances are constantly disrupted. Even if the losses and gains are not particularly large, they place the body under tremendous stress, as its physiological systems are overburdened with having to change, adjust, and adapt—again and again and again. Without question, the polymorph—whether he is slightly or excessively overweight—would be better off if he lost his excess pounds *permanently.*

CALORIES DO COUNT

No discussion of the physiology of overweight would be complete without some mention of calories. Even so, I feel somewhat uncomfortable discussing them. After all, the major thrust of my program has little to do with counting calories. My emphasis, instead, is on helping you understand and control your compulsive overeating. Although you will be eating sensibly and will probably be consuming fewer calories, counting calories should not be a major focus of your attention.

But to complete this chapter on the physiological aspects of polymorphism, let me briefly explain the mechanics of weight gain and loss. A *calorie* is nothing more than a measure of food energy. If you were to add an additional 3500 calories to your diet each week, you would become one pound fatter, assuming your body did not expend this energy in its normal daily functioning. Conversely, if you consumed 3500 fewer calories per week—or 500 fewer per day—you would lose a pound in that week.

Because of the many complicated physiological and psychological aspects of his disease, the compulsive overeater may find it more difficult to limit his caloric intake. He also has more fat cells that are eager to absorb any excess fat in his body. Even so, the basic process itself is identical in both fat and thin people—a reduction in calories means a reduction in weight. That's why a sensible eating plan is so important to your long-term success.

As arduous as your weight-loss task may seem now, you *can* reduce successfully, even if you have failed dozens of times before. Although I don't know you personally, of course, I know the intricacies of your disease. In my clinical experience, people suffering from the same compulsive overeating syndrome have been helped. In the next chapter, we will begin discussing your partner in detail. He or she will become the most important component in your own management of polymorphism.

4

The Vital Difference: A Mutual-Support System

After years of treating polymorphs, I am convinced that this no-diet, partnership-support program can finally offer you an effective approach to permanent weight loss. Unlike the diets you've tried in the past, the simple eating plan I will suggest will become part of your life, without being boring, impractical, or health-threatening with the passage of time. Instead, it will teach you to develop a more normal relationship to food, with the encouragement and support of a friend who can help you understand why you overeat and how you can finally lose weight for good. And the relationship is completely reciprocal—that is, you will provide the same support and encouragement for your partner that he or she provides for you.

Although this partner system may be entirely new to you, the concept is not revolutionary. I have personally served as a consultant for many self-help organizations over the last ten years. In 1971, after writing and presenting a paper on the status and effectiveness of self-help groups to the national conference of the American Psychiatric Association, I began advising and motivating many assemblages of people who share a common set of circumstances, from overeaters to alcoholics.

When people have a similar problem, they are better able to provide each other with caring and insights than any professional. True, I think it's important for each individual to assume responsibility for his own behavior. But when peers who are having similar experiences and feelings can communicate their genuine interest and concern, they can become extremely valuable in motivating others to change their own behavior. The well-documented success of organizations like Overeaters Anonymous and Alcoholics Anonymous shows how significant unconditional, day-by-day support can be. And in my own experience with overweight people, I have found that once they realize that they are not alone in their predicament, and that they are "normal" in spite of their excess weight and their insecurities, they abandon their feelings of helplessness, stop using food for solace, and finally start relying on themselves to alter their negative eating habits.

Over the next ten weeks, one of your partner's most important functions will be to make you consciously aware of the psychological factors related to how and why you eat. Most of the activities suggested in this program are designed to help you do just that. Also, in addition to developing an eating plan together, you will implement exercise and relaxation programs and talk to each other daily for support and encouragement.

As you'll learn in the upcoming weeks, a friend—a fellow polymorph—can be more helpful than an internist, psychiatrist, or psychologist who has a dozen degrees. True, your partner can't offer you the professional expertise and complex insights of a trained therapist. But as many studies have shown, he can offer you qualities that are essential to boost your self-esteem and change your relationship with food—namely, he can share his humanness, his genuine day-to-day concern, his closeness, his reason, his mutual problems, and his approachability. The self-help movement—and this no-diet program—owe their success to these very important human characteristics.

SELECTING A PARTNER

If you haven't already done so, I'd like you to begin thinking now about choosing a partner to work with in this ten-week program. Like many other people, your first reaction might be, "I'd rather do it on my own. If I put my mind to it, I know I can lose weight by myself." Unfortunately, we're taught in this society to believe that it's a weakness to ask for help, to be in a dependent position. But in reality, it takes much more strength to admit, "I need some help." After years of trying, you *haven't* been able to lose weight permanently on your own. Many people are now recognizing that they can benefit from some peer support. All I'm asking you to do is try it.

You can probably already think of a few people whom you might approach to become your partner for the next ten weeks—a friend, a neighbor, or a co-worker. When some polymorphs begin this program, they have difficulty deciding which of several friends to invite in as their partner. If that is your dilemma, you are very fortunate, and my advice is that you approach them all. If your group consists of three, four, five or more people—instead of only two—the support system will be even stronger. In such cases, you will break up into pairs (or a group of three if there's an odd number of people) to perform the exercises in this book, and then return to the larger group to discuss what you have learned. In almost all cases, the larger the group, the better.

Whether you decide upon one or several partners, the guidelines below will help you make your selection.

General Guidelines for Selecting a Partner

1. Your partner should have a weight problem. Although theoretically you could go through this program with a nonpolymorph, it's unlikely that the experience would be as ef-

fective. One of the foundations of the ten-week plan involves sharing thoughts and feelings with which your partner can easily identify. Someone who does not eat compulsively can't comprehend your predicament nearly as well as someone who does. Your partner, incidentally, need not have the same amount of weight to lose as you.

2. Your partner should be sincerely interested in losing weight. Some polymorphs, having failed so often on so many different diets, have simply given up and resigned themselves to being overweight. You need a person who, after reading this book, is willing to make a firm, ten-week commitment to ending his compulsive overeating.

3. Your partner should be someone you feel close to, someone with whom you can communicate freely and honestly. Do not select a person whom you feel you must impress or to whom you would feel uncomfortable admitting your imperfections.

4. Your partner should not be judgmental. Don't select someone you know in advance is likely to criticize everything you say or offer advice on "the best way" for you to behave.

5. Your partner should be someone who will be available to you not only for the scheduled biweekly meetings and daily phone calls, but also for hastily convened get-togethers during periods of "crisis."

6. Your partner should *not* be your spouse, parent, or other family member. Although husbands and wives sometimes can be successful partners, I don't recommend it. It's difficult for spouses to go through this program together, simply because of all the normal interpersonal conflicts and issues within every family. Sharing your feelings about the family interactions that may cause you to overeat can sometimes provoke a mate or other family member into a defensive or argumentative posture. Consequently, husbands and wives (as well as other close relatives)

are frequently unable to provide the kind of support the polymorph needs to make progress, to move forward.

This last point needs some amplification. My clinical research shows that, subconsciously, a spouse may occasionally want his or her mate to stay fat for a variety of reasons. Spouses are sometimes afraid that their mates, upon becoming thin, will develop new friendships, and a new social life that might exclude them. Some husbands and wives are subconsciously anxious about a thinner mate becoming more attractive to the opposite sex or making greater sexual demands, perhaps resulting in an extramarital affair or other disruptions in the relationship. One man admitted, "Whenever my wife was on a diet, I used to say to her, 'Just a little piece of candy isn't going to hurt' or 'Take a break from your diet; you can go back on it tomorrow.'" Although these are all generally unconscious conflicts in the spouse, they further undermine the polymorph's ability to cope with his problem.

In order to stop eating compulsively and lose weight for good, you need a friend or confidant who has been there like you have, who will have more of an understanding without a personal stake in your remaining a polymorph. Your partner can offer you something your family can't—a safe, nonthreatening environment where value judgments and histories won't be a part of your relationship.

Family members should be kept informed of the progress of the program. However, the interaction between you and your partner will be something special that could confuse family members or make them feel left out. To prevent that from happening, apprise them often of the value you're deriving from the program, and let them know that in the ninth week you'll bring them in to help you carry your new insights, behavior, and weight loss into the future.

Having eliminated family members from your list of potential partners, it's time to approach one or more of the friends and fellow polymorphs you have in mind. You might just say something as simple as "I've been reading a book about a ten-week, no-diet program that sounds exciting. I'd like to give it to you to read. When you're finished, let's talk about it." Or you can try piquing a friend's interest by observing, "If you're as tired of diets as I am, let me tell you about this new program. It's a no-diet plan for weight loss, and I think it'd be fun to do together." Or, "This book is based on a partner system for losing weight that seems like it will work; do you want to try it?"

Whatever words you use, make a determined effort to find yourself someone with whom to share this experience. The mutual-support system is your key to permanent weight loss. You must find a partner willing to commit himself to the program and to communicate effectively with you. Fortunately, there is a vast psychological literature on proper communication, sensitive listening, and successful peer counseling. In the remainder of this chapter, I will discuss what I feel are the most effective techniques for you and your partner to use to support one another in the no-diet program.

THE ART OF BEING A PARTNER

Communicating Openly

This program has been reshaped and streamlined several times, based on how patients have responded to it. But one element has remained stable: the necessity for open and honest communication between you and your partner. Throughout the ten weeks, I will provide topics for the two of you to discuss and some specific questions that will get the dialogue started. But it is up to you to talk as sincerely and candidly as possible.

This kind of straightforward sharing may sound difficult to achieve. Almost everyone is embarrassed at first to talk about their abuse of food or the emotional difficulties that may be causing them to overeat. Polymorphs are convinced that no one else in the world secretly binges or eats to escape from their worries. They imagine that they will be ridiculed or disliked if they admit to such behavior. They believe they're supposed to be perfect.

We all set impossible standards of perfection for ourselves. We forget that everyone has flaws and even the people we admire most make mistakes. Once you and your partner can acknowledge your wish to be "perfect" to one another, most of your embarrassment will disappear. As I will repeat throughout this book, your partner has had many of the same eating—and life—experiences as you. You won't find yourself being judged or laughed at. In fact, in professionally observing the interactions of people for many years, I have found that someone will usually like you *more* once you are willing to share yourself openly with them. And you'll probably find yourselves laughing together over the experience.

Maryann was terribly apprehensive the day she told her partner, "I did the most disgusting thing last night. I'm sure you've never done this, but I have to tell you about it. I took a pint of ice cream to bed, and ate two-thirds of it before I put it away." But Maryann's anxiety quickly disappeared when her friend laughed, "I just ate a quart!" They were both relieved to discover that their behavior wasn't so unusual, after all. And it opened up the communication channels for months of candid sharing. You'll find that your fears will self-destruct as soon as you and your partner begin to talk with each other.

As one woman told me, "The moment I trusted my partner, I got more gratification than from all the meals I could ever eat. I started thinking about things other than eating for the first time in years. Food finally became only something to fulfill my nutritional requirements. I found myself eating less, without even trying hard."

In the upcoming weeks, as you begin to communicate openly and discuss, for example, the negative impact of compulsive overeating on your life, you'll receive such positive feelings (professionals call them "secondary gains") from this communication that you'll be less likely to resort to overeating for comfort. And even if you do backslide, your partner will be there to support and stabilize you until even stronger, more positive patterns take hold.

Listening Effectively

You and your partner can assist one another in communicating effectively by refining your own listening skills. Listening is more than just absorbing sound waves; it requires one's thorough and undivided attention. Unfortunately, few people really listen well; instead, most of us are thinking about what we are going to say next, waiting for an opportunity to jump in. Or we activate our mind's sorting apparatus and don't really hear everything that others are saying, instead filtering and evaluating what is being said based on past experiences and judgments.

To maximize your effectiveness as a partner, you need to know how to listen properly. You will have to devote yourself not only to hearing your friend's words but to discerning the tone of his voice and observing his facial expressions in order to help discover what he really is *feeling*. In this program, feelings are as important as thoughts, and you owe it to your partner to be sensitive to them. By helping each other get in touch with and organize your feelings and emotions, you will gain insight into why you compulsively overeat.

The principles of "active listening" are simple to follow, and have proven very helpful for polymorphs in this program:

1. Seat yourself directly opposite your partner so that you are positioned face to face. Lean slightly forward to involve yourself completely in the experience, and make eye contact with the other person.

2. Give your partner your total attention by setting aside your own reactions to what is being said and allowing only the substance of his words to occupy your mind. Your skills at focusing your concentration this way will become more sophisticated with time.

3. Take notice of his tone of voice and his facial expressions, which often communicate the feelings underlying his verbal message.

During these ten weeks, you may find that you are hearing and feeling more from another person than ever before in your life. Fortunately, the communication skills you are learning here can be integrated into your daily relationships with people forever, making your life more fulfilling long after the ten weeks are over.

Responding Constructively

Learning how to respond constructively is as important for effective communication as active listening. A constructive and appropriate response to your partner does not involve giving advice; rather, it entails helping your partner formulate, understand, and interpret his own thoughts and feelings and then decide for himself the most appropriate action he can take. You and your partner, better than anyone else, will each eventually define and explain your own personal behavior and motivations. You are there primarily as sounding boards for one another, to gently encourage and support each other as you sift through your respective experiences.

Of course, it's human nature to want to give advice. Linda, for example, was aghast when she received a call from her partner announcing that she was about to devour a box of chocolates. "My first instinct was to say, 'Stop! Don't do that!'" Linda recalls. "But then I recognized that I was trying to control her behavior which wasn't the best thing I could do for her.

The only thing I could control was my own behavior. So I simply said, 'Tell me about it.' We started talking, and she began to describe the anxieties that had built up during the day, which had pushed her close to finding comfort in some chocolates. We talked for almost an hour, and she finally decided on her own that she didn't want or need the candy after all."

As a partner, your obligation is to encourage your friend to take responsibility for his own problems and actions. He has the knowledge and ability to arrive at conclusions in his own best interest once you provide the vehicle to sort out his feelings, needs, and desires in relation to food. If your partner wants to binge, your task is to help guide him toward exploring the feelings that are causing such urges. He won't make any progress if you stand beside him shouting, "Don't do it!" But if you allow him to take responsibility for his own situation—just as he will do for you—you are telling him, in effect, "I respect your ability to figure things out for yourself. I'm here to assist you in doing that, but not to do it for you."

Below are some important principles for constructive responding that you and your partner should familiarize yourselves with before the ten-week program begins:

1. In order to avoid giving advice, refrain from using sentences that contain words like "should" or "ought." For instance:

> "You ought to stop buying ice cream to tempt you every time you open the freezer."
>
> "You should tell your spouse to stop pestering you about your weight."
>
> Your partner is quite capable of solving his own problems and making his own decisions. Let him do so.

2. Try not to be judgmental in your responses to what your partner says or does. If you criticize or assail his eating behaviors or other actions, you will only create anxiety, tension,

and frustration in him. If your partner is telling you how his poor self-image is causing him to overeat, he doesn't need you to say, "You're silly to feel that way" or "When are you going to get off this self-deprecating soapbox?" He is telling you how he's misusing food. If you respond constructively (see specific techniques below), he will eventually begin really listening to what he's saying, and investigating possible solutions to his problem.

Thus, the best course is to allow any personal judgments to pass through your mind without verbalizing them. Once your partner feels that he can be open and honest with you, without any possibility of being attacked, there is a far better chance of his objectively exploring with you all of his alternatives out of his predicament.

3. The most effective way to help your partner listen to himself is to rephrase his statements in as accurate a portrayal of what he says as possible. Act as a mirror, letting him hear the content of his own remarks in an original way. Begin these reflections with phrases like, "What you seem to be saying is that ———," or "In other words, ———." For example, "What you seem to be saying is that food has been a substitute for a lot of things missing in your life" or "In other words, you really believe that your family has never been supportive in helping you lose weight." This will assist your friend in clarifying his own thoughts and give him a springboard from which to continue the discussion.

4. When appropriate, help your partner define what he is *feeling*. You can often do this by trying to put yourself in his place ("What would I be feeling right now if I were saying the things that Cheryl is saying?") Then simply express your reaction in a brief sentence to your partner. For example:

"If that happened to me, I would feel angry."

"If that happened to me, I would feel happy."

"If that happened to me, I would feel depressed."

"If that happened to me, I would feel confused."

Sometimes, you can help your partner define *why* he is feeling the way he is, just by extending the sentence a few words:

"I would feel angry if someone had been treating me like a child ever since I gained weight."

"I would feel pleased by making an unwavering commitment to this no-diet program."

"I would feel unhappy with myself if I had been unable to develop a meaningful relationship with my mother."

When done effectively, this technique will provide your partner with some additional input with which to examine his life situation.

5. When you sense that your partner hasn't fully clarified a particular issue, your job is to ask questions to help him further explore the matter at hand. You can often do this by *sharing related experiences of your own* or by attaching a question to one of the above statements. For example:

"How exactly have people treated you like a child since your weight gain?"

"Why did you decide to make a commitment to this no-diet program now?"

His answers to such questions will add even further depth to his self-exploration.

6. Communicate your concern and caring toward your partner. Let him know that you're trying to understand the world as he sees it and that you want to help him, in whatever way he feels most comfortable, to lose weight permanently and improve the quality of his life. If you truly care, and can communicate this caring to your partner, you will have done your job.

An essential element of this program is your genuine commitment to be responsive to and supportive of your partner at all times. As the two of you discuss the issues that will be raised in the next ten weeks, your respective functions are to help each other clarify the thoughts and feelings underlying what is said. Before either of you can make any permanent changes in your eating behavior, a clear sense must exist of the problems that are present and of the options that are available.

PART 2

THE TEN-WEEK NO-DIET PROGRAM

THIS TEN-WEEK NO-DIET PROGRAM, WHICH I HAVE already briefly described, is probably unlike any other weight-loss plan you've ever encountered. With your partner, you'll be exploring and sharing your histories and attitudes concerning your compulsive overeating. You'll be talking about the anxieties, frustrations, and failures surrounding your chronic inability to lose weight.

This program promises gradual and permanent weight loss. Medical research is certain about one thing: the only healthy way to achieve long-lasting weight reduction is *slowly*. You may be impatient now for instant results. But if you are willing to commit yourself to a ten-week program, you will achieve long-term results that no quick-weight-loss scheme has ever provided.

Once you've chosen a friend to accompany you through this no-diet approach, you're ready to get started. There are just a few basic ground rules for you to follow.

1. *Make a promise to meet twice a week for ten weeks.* Each meeting should last at least sixty minutes, although many polymorphs extend the sessions to ninety minutes to get as much out of the program as possible. I suggest that you always schedule your meetings on the same two days each week (for example, every Monday and Thursday at 5:00, or every Tuesday and Friday at 9:00) to help establish a regular routine. Try to make certain that neither of you will have any conflicting appointments on those days to interfere with your meetings.

Agree now to stick with the program for ten full weeks. As I've said, this program has been designed with *permanent* weight loss as its goal. It will take you the full ten weeks to begin to establish new, lasting patterns of eating behavior. Approach it *one day at a time*, and the new habits you'll learn will soon become a satisfying part of your life.

2. *Hold each meeting in a comfortable, quiet, private place,* free of distractions and noise. Most people choose their homes as the most appropriate meeting places, but if you have a spouse and/or children try to schedule your sessions when they aren't at home. This is a private time for you and your partner, an opportunity to concentrate on nothing but yourselves. You'll soon find that you really look forward to these meetings, so do what you can to minimize interruptions during your sessions. The payoff will be worth the extra effort.

3. *Follow the program sequentially.* Don't submit to the temptation to jump ahead. You may feel like speed-reading your way through the book and grappling with only those areas that seem most relevant to you. While I have no objection to your reading ahead, don't perform any of the activities out of order or delete any of them. This program must be *experienced,* as well as intellectually understood. At times, I'm certain you'll say to yourself or your partner, "I've got that; I know what he's trying to say. What's next?" But you will get the full value of the program only by going through each activity in its what he's trying to say. What's next?" But you will get the vull value of the program only by going through each activity in its proper sequence. Each meeting builds upon the insights you've gained in previous ones, so follow the instructions and proceed in order, from day to day and week to week.

"This plan is not like waving a magic wand," observed one patient recently. "All of my weight didn't fall off overnight, and there was some rough going along the way. But I took it step by step, and gradually became aware of what had been going on with my eating and how I could change it. It took time, but it worked."

This program is extremely successful for people who are willing to follow its guidelines.

THE ELEMENTS OF THE PROGRAM

The Regular Biweekly Meetings

As you've learned, the twice-a-week meetings with your partner are critical elements in this program. During these meetings, you will discuss issues relevant to your polymorphism and your control of it. After the first couple of sessions, every meeting will include a self-evaluation of your progress. Also, during each session, you will practice a regular exercise regimen and relaxation technique. You will learn some simple behavior-modification activities, designed to make you consciously aware of food and how you relate to it, which will help you alter negative eating habits. You and your partner will have many discussions about the important people in your lives (including parents, spouses, and children) and how your interactions with them may be influencing your eating habits. You'll also evaluate your self-esteem and try to determine if you are punishing yourself by overeating or using food as a tranquilizer to escape from stress and anxiety.

These are all important parts of the ten-week program, and each will be reinforced by the encouragement, support, and participation of your partner.

The Calling-in Plan and Your Daily Menu

Every day, you and your friend will independently decide what you will eat for the next twenty-four hours, and you will call and share that menu with each other. This system is designed to put each of you in command of your own eating behavior, rather than letting you be manipulated by food.

With the nutritional guidelines I will suggest, you will each have decided in advance what you will eat that day—three reasonable, well-balanced meals—and, once having committed yourself to this menu by calling it in to your partner, you'll find that you won't be nearly as tempted to deviate. But when you do think you can't control the impulse—and *everyone* feels that way from time to time—you will learn to call your partner for encouragement and moral support. Over time, as the two of you begin to deal more normally with food, you will gradually start to lose weight.

You probably are still trying to figure out, calculate, and intellectualize precisely *how* this program can work. For the present, you need not understand every process thoroughly, but just be willing to accept it. As a growing number of polymorphs have learned, sharing and exploring their fears, depression, anxiety, loneliness, and other experiences can mark the beginning of the weight-loss process. Withhold your own judgment for a while, and soon you will sense that something is changing. Before long, you will have begun to lose weight—permanently.

Week 1

DAY 1

NINE "GOOD" REASONS FOR POSTPONING THE FIRST MEETING

"I had a fight with my husband/wife/lover."

"My child is having trouble in school."

"My kitchen is being remodeled, but we'll start as soon as it's done."

"I can't lose weight during summer when there are so many other things to do."

"I'm being audited by the IRS."

"I twisted my ankle."

"I have extra responsibilities at the office because my coworker is on maternity leave."

"I'm working nights."

"My sister is getting married this month, and I have to do all the planning."

Above are a few of the excuses and rationalizations that I've heard from polymorphs who had anxieties about beginning this program. Some may sound ridiculous, but to the person saying them, they're real. Have you thought of a few excuses of your own?

Let me reassure you that if you are feeling nervous about getting started for any reason, that is all right. Almost everyone does. It's completely natural. Simply start by acknowledging it aloud. Discuss it with your partner and ask him if he is feeling any such resistances. Sharing your thoughts will begin the process of opening communication.

This program can work for every polymorph, no matter what your resistances. But you have to give it a chance. This initial sixty-to-ninety-minute meeting with your partner is the first step.

Even if you and your partner have already known each other for several months or even years, it is likely that you have never discussed some of the intimate subjects that form the basis of this program—for example, your private eating behavior, thoughts and feelings about being overweight, or your self-image and self-esteem. In a week or two, though, once you recognize how many attitudes the two of you have in common, any anxiety you may feel now about communicating candidly will disappear.

Many polymorphs are anxious about starting this program for another reason—namely, they dread beginning still another weight-loss program, having failed with so many in the past. Understandably, they simply don't want to fail again. As one woman said, "The thought of getting my hopes up to lose weight, only to gain it all back again, makes me miserable. I want to lose weight, and I'm intrigued by this no-diet program, but I'm also a little nervous about being disappointed again."

In addition, some people may feel tense about starting this program for what is probably a wholly unconscious reason—the "secondary gains" they receive from their excess weight. That is, people treat them in ways they consider desirable because they are polymorphs. For example, if your friends are compassionate toward you because of your weight, you might unconsciously want to remain obese rather than relinquish this attention from others. Or your excess weight may permit you to avoid sexual encounters or social responsibilities.

"When I was overweight, I think it disgusted my husband," recalled Lois. "We stopped making love, which I never really enjoyed anyway. Looking back, I guess I knew that as long as I stayed fat, I could avoid having sex with him. And so although I went through the motions of starting diets every now and then, I don't think I ever really wanted to lose the weight. But in my discussions with my partner, I finally realized that my behavior—and my overweight problem—were hurting only me. I finally decided to change."

To begin this ten-week program, discuss any resistances you may be feeling, which may stand between you and complete success with this no-diet plan. You must recognize what they are before you can eventually overcome them.

Today, as in every other day of the program, I will ask you and your partner to participate in various activities together, each of which plays an important role in attaining permanent weight loss. So let's get started. Open yourself up to this program—and to your partner—and approach it one day at a time.

TAKING PHOTOGRAPHS

To begin this first session, I want you and your partner to take full-length photographs of one another, fully clothed. So bring a camera (not a Polaroid) with you. After you have each taken a shot or two, remove the film from the camera, but don't send it to the drugstore or camera shop for developing. Simply take the photographs and put the film away.

In a couple of months, I'll ask you to process the film

and, in the tenth week of the program, to compare the "old" photographs with the "new" you. The pictures will be proof of your progress, and will have an even greater psychological impact than the number of pounds you have lost.

WEIGHING AND MEASURING

Next, you and your partner will weigh and measure one another, and record the results on the Weights and Measurements chart shown below. (You'll need to make a second copy of the chart so both of you will have one.) Use a tape measure, and systematically determine the size of the chest/bust, upper arms, waist, hips, thighs, and calves. First, you should measure your partner, and then he should measure you.

There may be some tension and nervousness in this process. After all, you are sharing intimate information about your body—information that you may have tried to conceal from others for years. But be willing to go through this procedure with your partner, even if you feel a little uncomfortable doing so. These meetings together are being held in a protected, nonthreatening, nonjudgmental environment where you can feel free to be yourself. By being honest with your partner about your size and weight, you will simultaneously bring this information into your own conscious awareness, allowing yourself, finally, to begin dealing with it realistically.

This chart will become an important part of your program, particularly if your weight should plateau at a certain level. At various times, you may stop losing literal weight, which can be terribly frustrating. But during these stages, your body may actually be redistributing your weight. You will see changes in your hips, waist, and other measurements, and people will ask you whether you've lost weight when you actually haven't. Be prepared for these plateaus; almost everyone experiences them. It's all part of the process.

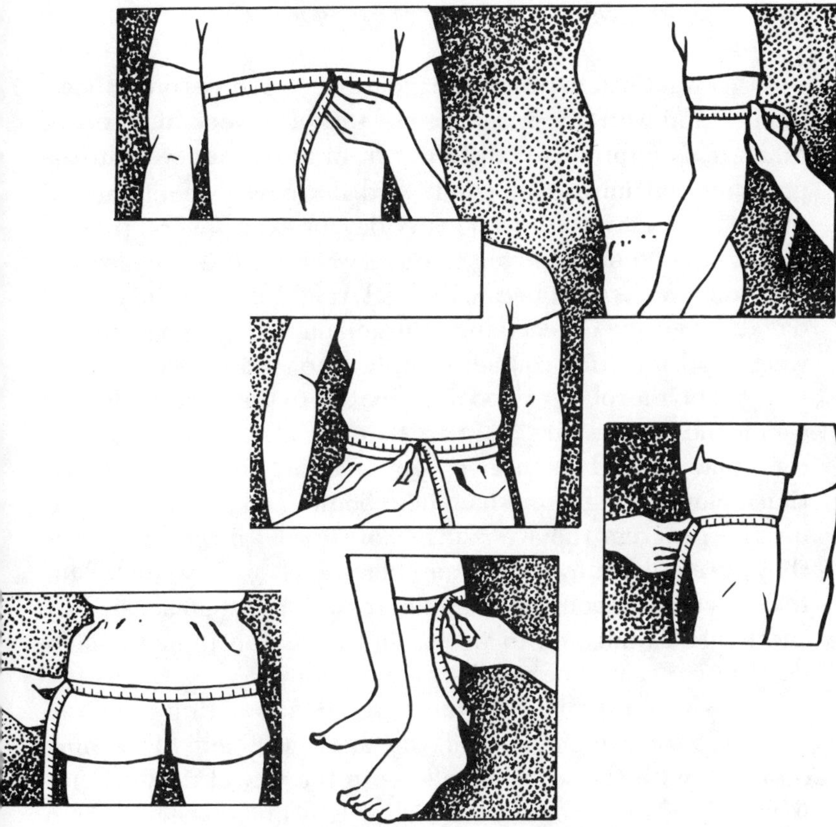

WEIGHTS AND MEASUREMENTS

	Week 1	Week 2	Week 3
Weight			
Chest (Bust)			
Biceps			
Waist			
Hips			
Thighs			
Calves			

I want you to weigh and measure yourselves only once a month. You won't do it again until the fifth week of this program. This approach is different from any other weight-loss program you have ever tried. And if you've become accustomed to weighing yourself every day, or even several times a day, it may seem agonizing to stay away from the scale for the next four weeks. But because actual weight loss can be unpredictable and even deceiving, I urge you and your partner to weigh and measure yourselves only when I ask you to.

Polymorphs give too much power to their scales. If they weigh themselves and discover that the program is working, they may reward themselves by deviating from their nutritional plan, eating more than they should, and thus undermining the progress they've made. Conversely, if they find that they *haven't* lost any weight, or not as much as they wanted to, they become discouraged and depressed, tell themselves that "nothing's ever going to work," and return to their old self-destructive eating behavior.

If you are following the program and eating properly, you *will* lose weight. But if you allow yourself to become obsessed with the scale, it will get in the way of dealing with issues like *why* you overeat, which will ultimately allow you to keep your excess weight off permanently.

"Until I started on this program, the scale ruled my life," recalls Mindy. "The first thing I'd do in the morning was weigh myself, and my mood for the day would be determined by my weight. If I was heavier than I thought I should be, I'd be depressed. If I had lost a pound, I'd be happy. But I eventually recognized that there were other things in life that could give me *genuine* happiness, including the people around me. Once I quit thinking about my weight all the time, I started losing it. And I've kept it off."

Although it may seem natural for you and your partner to set weight-loss goals, I would like you to refrain from this practice as well. Everyone, of course, has an idea of how much weight they would like to lose. But like frequent weighing, goals can sabotage a reducing program. If you attain your goal, you will feel like your objective has been reached and thus abandon the program. As soon as you do, you will begin gaining back the weight. By contrast, if it appears that you aren't reaching your goal, you may become frustrated, conclude that the program is not working, and start eating compulsively again.

So even though you probably already know how much weight you would like to lose, try not to allow yourself to become preoccupied with a number. This program is carefully designed for gradual and permanent results. Although well-meaning family and friends may ask you how much weight you've lost, short-term indications really don't count. Rather, by adhering to this program, you'll experience a trend toward weight loss that will become lifelong.

DISCUSSING TODAY'S MEETING

Now, I want you and your partner to seat yourselves opposite one another and begin one of many discussions that you will have together in the next ten weeks. This particular dialogue should last only perhaps ten minutes, with the purpose being primarily to make yourselves comfortable exchanging ideas with one another.

Before you begin, you might turn back to Chapter 4 and quickly review the guidelines for communicating effectively. If you adhere to the techniques described there, you and your partner will both find yourselves communicating more openly, thanks to the honesty and encouragement you are offering one another.

Use the suggested topics below as possible springboards for your discussion today:

1. In general, how do you feel today, beginning this program with your partner? Excited? Nervous? Skeptical? Eager? Discuss the thoughts that both of you have as you enter this program.

2. How did you each feel about weighing and measuring one another? Were you more (less) anxious than you had expected? In general, discuss your reactions to confronting your actual weight and measurements and revealing them to someone else.

3. Do you feel uncomfortable about weighing yourself only once a month? Do you expect to have difficulty staying away from the scale? Discuss with your partner what might be the benefits related to such infrequent weigh-ins.

4. Are you both agreeable to the absence of weight-loss goals in this program? Discuss the reasons that goals can be detrimental.

Spend a few minutes talking about the topics that seem relevant and interesting, allowing your partner to help you define and consolidate your thoughts and feelings.

TALKING ABOUT YOUR PARENTS

For the next twenty to twenty-five minutes, I want you and your partner to each talk about your own parents, sharing your feelings about how you see them in relation to you. Initially, this may seem unconnected to the polymorph syndrome and losing weight. But, as you will recall from the introductory chapters, your self-esteem can play a major role in not only weight gain but also permanent weight loss. Psychiatrists and psychologists agree without question that your parents and their feelings toward you are often important contributing factors in the status of your self-esteem and your overweight problem. They are not the only factors, but may play a major role.

Consider the images of yourself that you received from your parents. You carry them around with you for your entire life, whether or not your parents are still living. And they affect your behavior and the way you feel about yourself. Once you start to talk about them, with the support and caring of your partner, you will begin easing the pent-up anxieties and stress that, until now, you may have tried to tranquilize with food.

So in order to understand your compulsive overeating better, and the feelings that may be affecting your behavior, start by discussing some of your feelings toward your parents. (At your next meeting, the discussion will switch to how your parents felt about *you*.) Each of you should take a turn speaking. Share your thoughts and feelings openly, talking about whatever might come to mind. To trigger your discussion, here are some questions that may get you started. You and your partner can ask them of one another, while also feeling free to explore any other areas that you would like to:

How did you feel about your father/mother?

Did your parents have a guiding attitude toward life?

How did they react during times of conflict or hardship?

What was their relationship with one another?

What did your parents argue about?

Did your parents have any particular anxieties or fears that they communicated to you, which may be influencing your behavior?

What did they usually talk about at the dinner table?

Did they treat your siblings differently from you?

If you could, how would you have changed your mother/father?

How would you characterize your mother's/father's attitude toward food and eating?

What is your overall impression of your parents?

Being completely open and honest with your partner may seem difficult at first. When Caroline's partner first asked her "How would you have changed your parents?" Caroline responded "Oh, I wouldn't change them. They did the best they could." But, referring to the guidelines for effective communication in Chapter 4, her partner helped her by rephrasing the question: "So they did their best. But what would you have liked to see different about them?" This time, Caroline's answer was more direct. "I just wish they had loved me more. I always felt that they loved my younger sister more than me, and gave her more attention, and thought she was prettier."

Caroline's perception of her parents' favoritism may have been mistaken. They may have loved and treated their daughters equally, as far as they were concerned. But that's not the way Caroline perceived it, and how she perceived it became her reality. Beginning with this discussion, she progressively learned to make peace with the parental images she had integrated into her own belief system. "If they do feel that way about me, that's okay. It's only their opinion. I'm just as worthy as my sister."

Once Caroline could begin talking candidly with her partner, she felt relieved and the words and feelings began to flow. That's a common experience. If you initially feel a thick wall between you and your partner, be willing to make the first move to crack it. When the two of you start sharing, it will become so rewarding that you may not want to stop. Once you start receiving comfort and love from a genuine source—another human being—you will stop filling yourself up with food. In fact, as Caroline's self-esteem progressively improved, she noticed that her need to use food to comfort or numb her feelings ebbed. She had finally started to successfully manage her compulsive overeating.

"When I talked with my partner, my past was no longer buried inside of me to gnaw at me anymore," recalled Harry. "I had spent most of my life denying my feelings. Once I put it out there and my partner and I looked at it, I realized for the first time that the past really wasn't so terrible. I really wasn't so bad, either. And almost automatically, I began to gain some control over my overeating."

Finally, don't expect you and your partner to arrive at any major life-changing conclusions today. This is only your first meeting. Your understanding of the polymorph syndrome will increase with each session and grow during the intervening days. But you have taken an important initial step toward controlling your compulsive overeating today.

AFFIRMING YOUR COMMITMENT

Before you conclude this first meeting, it is important for you and your partner to make a firm commitment to continue these sessions together regularly, twice a week for ten weeks. There is a growing "synergistic" effect that occurs when you meet regularly—the content of each meeting builds upon and reinforces the experiences of the last one. If you start finding reasons not to meet, there could be many *subconscious* reasons why. As I've suggested, perhaps you're afraid of failing at this program. Maybe you have a wish not to deny yourself food. Or part of you may not want to give up those secondary gains—attention, comfort, freedom from social demands—that I talked about earlier. These are issues that you should discuss with your partner as you begin to recognize them.

This no-diet program offers you an alternative to the problematic aspects of your life that influence your behavior.

But it can work for you only with a serious commitment on your part to follow the guidelines week by week and come to the scheduled meetings. In fact, I would like you and your partner to sign a contract with one another, affirming your intention to meet regularly during the ten-week program. It need not be complicated, merely saying something like this:

> I, (your name) ________________,
> and I, (your partner's name) ________________,
> pledge to meet together every Monday and Thursday, from 10:00 to 11:00 A.M., for the next ten weeks to carry out the no-diet program.
>
> Signed,
>
> ________________
>
> ________________
>
> ________________
>
> Date

I recognize that the idea of a contract may seem artificial to you. One woman complained, "I said I'm coming to the meetings. Why do I have to sign this?" But as silly as it may appear, the written agreement will make your commitment stronger. Signing the contract will carry more power than a verbal pact. A commitment on paper will make it more difficult for you to retreat from the program during the moments of doubt and apprehension that everyone experiences.

Fortunately, such misgivings eventually disappear for most people. One polymorph recently told me that the time spent with her partner quickly became some of the most important and enjoyable moments of her week. It was a special time just for her and her friend, with no outside demands being made upon them. Your meetings are just for the two of you (or for all of you if your group consists of three or more). That's one of the reasons they work.

DAY 2

EVALUATING YOUR PROGRESS

To begin your second meeting with your partner, spend a few minutes discussing the previous meeting and the intervening days. What have your thoughts and feelings been? Do you feel any resistance about continuing the program or coming to the meetings? Did you weigh yourself, or did you successfully stay away from the scale the past few days? Has it been difficult for you to avoid setting weight-loss goals? Have you had any other ideas about how your parents might have influenced your polymorphism?

You and your partner should take turns discussing these and any other issues on your mind. This dialogue may last only five minutes or it could extend much longer. Take as much time as necessary to talk about what has gone on in your mind or in your life thus far.

Listen to what your partner has to say. Encourage each other to be as open and specific as possible. The warmth and support you give each other greatly affects how much benefit you'll both gain from the program.

THE FOOD DIARY

To continue this meeting, I'd like you and your friend to examine the Food Diary below. Make several copies of the diary, for you and your partner to use to keep a record of everything you eat between this meeting and the next.

This chart is an important part of this ten-week program. It will provide you with a profile of your eating behavior, which will ultimately help you change *how* you eat. There are many variables in your environment (family members, emotions, activities, etc.) that determine and condition your habits relative to food. This chart will help you recognize exactly why you eat as you do, as the first step to changing your negative eating behaviors.

Look over the Food Diary with your partner. As you'll see, in addition to space for noting what, when, where, and how much you ate, you'll also indicate your mood during that particular meal or snack. For example, each time you eat, you'll ask yourself whether you are bored. Or are you depressed? Happy? Fatigued? Also, note any events that may have influenced your mood—for example, a conflict with your mate/child/parent, your boss making unfair demands on you, your son or daughter dating someone whom you disapprove of. And how long did it take you to eat, who prepared the meal, whom did you eat with, and what other activities were you engaged in while eating?

From now until your next meeting, jot down the appropriate information each time you eat, using a new sheet each day. It should take no more than a few seconds. Keep the Food Diary in your purse or pocket, where it will be easily accessible so that you won't be tempted not to use it.

Try to avoid altering your eating patterns over the next few days as you keep your diary, because changing your normal pattern will defeat the whole purpose of clearly seeing what your relationship with food really is. You want to determine what your problem areas are, so write down everything you eat, including second helpings and snacks—and be *honest*.

By keeping the Food Diary, one polymorph discovered that she snacked primarily when she was tired. Whenever fatigue set in, she was prone to a binge. Another polymorph found that he ate when he wanted to relax ("During coffee breaks, I would have two or three doughnuts; it was as much a part of relaxing as loosening my tie"). Still another ate whenever she felt lonely. Other polymorphs tell me that they overeat during periods of anger, frustration, shyness, sexual tension, and boredom ("I don't know what else to do until dinnertime, so I eat").

FOOD DIARY

DATE:		Mood							Foods and Amounts				
	Time												
	Start	End	Depressed	Bored	Happy	Fatigued	Excited	Angry	Other	(small, medium, or large serving)	Who Prepared the Food	Eaten Alone or with Whom	Exact Place Where Eaten	Associated Activities While Eating (e.g., reading, cooking, talking)
Breakfast														
Midmorning														
Lunch														
Afternoon														
Dinner														
After dinner														
Before bedtime														

Events of the day that could influence mood or eating:

Physical activities of the day:

The purpose of the Food Diary, again, is to make you consciously aware of your eating behavior, and of the emotions and activities that accompany your eating. Not only are the polymorph's actions dictated by psychological forces and images that may date back to childhood (like parental attitudes), but they are also controlled simply by habit. You may have conditioned yourself to eat particular foods at certain times without ever realizing it. These eating habits have evolved outside of your conscious awareness; they have become compulsive behaviors.

Once you recognize these habits—and your partner may be able to help you discover even more of them—this ten-week program will help you create your own well-defined eating plan to counteract them. You will also be introduced to other activities to teach you new, more positive behaviors in place of the negative ones. With your partner's help, you will begin reconditioning yourself, ultimately changing your eating patterns for good.

After you've examined the Food Diary with your partner, discuss aloud what you think some of your negative eating behaviors might be. Do either of you, for instance, eat when you are cooking? Driving? After scolding the children, or following an argument with a friend or your spouse? Do you eat with other people, or by yourself? Under what other circumstances do you overeat? Also discuss any anxiety, embarrassment or discomfort you may have concerning your Food Diary. Be aware of those feelings, but don't let them alter your commitment to the program. Your partner probably shares many of the eating habits you do, and the apprehensions will disappear as you discuss them.

TALKING ABOUT PARENTS

Next, let's return to the discussion of your parents that you and your partner began at the first meeting. As you did then, feel free to move the conversation in any direction you wish, with the guideline this time of focusing upon how your parents felt about *you*, and the messages they communicated to you. You and your partner should take turns talking about your own parental relationship, with each partner offering guidance and support. If your friend is having trouble defining the feelings that are accompanying his thoughts, you can help him by silently asking yourself, "What would I be feeling right now if I were saying the things he is?" Then express your reaction aloud to your partner (for example, "I would feel angry if my father did that"). This will help him understand as clearly as possible his attitudes and emotions.

The following questions are intended to help stimulate this conversation about parents, but feel free to use any of your own as well:

How did your father/mother compliment you? What would he/she say and do?

How did your father/mother criticize you? What would he/she say or do?

What did your father/mother forbid you to do?

What did your father/mother encourage you to do?

What general attitudes did your father/mother give you about life, about other people, about work, and about money?

What did your father/mother tell you about the opposite sex and marriage?

How would your father/mother describe you?

In a discussion with her partner, Diana recalled that her father, in a fit of anger, once told her, "You're no good; you're worthless." Even though this outburst was an isolated incident, she never forgot it. And it continued to have such an enormous impact upon her emotional well-being and her self-esteem that it may have become an influence on her overeating.

"I've always felt that I had to prove to my father that I'm okay," Diana told her partner. "But whenever I do something wrong—even get a traffic ticket—I can't help feeling maybe he was right." Her partner identified immediately with these feelings. She, too, had some lingering impressions of unworthiness left over from childhood. Diana and her partner ultimately realized that, as a way of quelling their anxieties that they were perhaps "not okay," they had learned to overeat.

During this discussion of parental attitudes, let me once again ask you to avoid being judgmental about anything your partner says. Be a good listener, not an advisor; a friend, not a parent. If you are judgmental ("How could you ever think something like that about your mom?"), your partner will probably become defensive rather than candid, and nothing meaningful will be learned. As a friend, you can help your partner focus specifically on the issues being discussed. Repeat questions that aren't answered directly. Rephrase what he is telling you to give him a clearer perspective on what he is feeling and thinking. In the process, you will both find that a tremendous amount of information will be related in just a few minutes.

While each of you talks, you both will realize that all those "terrible" feelings about your parents that you had never planned to tell anyone aren't so dreadful and unusual, after all. After these feelings are spoken, you can finally begin dealing with concrete issues rather than abstract feelings. If you and your partner can understand, accept, and begin to resolve the conflicts in your life in the upcoming weeks, you may no longer feel a need to overeat as a way of tranquilizing yourself against anxieties.

ANTICIPATING TRANSITIONS

In the next few weeks, you will be experiencing many new feelings about yourself. And as you begin to lose weight, you will notice behavioral changes occurring and emotions surfacing, some of which may be difficult to deal with. You will be experiencing emotional transitions, and coping with them will be easier if you and your partner know what to expect.

At some time in their life, many polymorphs deny that they even have an overweight problem. They become so afraid of confronting the compulsive nature of the polymorph syndrome that, for a while, it's easier to pretend it doesn't exist. Some polymorphs become depressed or even angry that they are overweight, with complaints like, "Why can other people eat so much more than me and not gain anything? It's not fair." Eventually, as you and your friend clearly recognize the compulsive component of your problem, you will grow more willing to explore your alternatives for change and accept responsibility for dealing with your overeating. Willingness to change and sensitivity to yourselves and each other are the keys to permanent weight loss.

Week 2

DAY 1

EVALUATING YOUR PROGRESS

To begin the second week, you and your partner should discuss any thoughts and feelings you have today about the program, yourselves, or your compulsive overeating. Because you haven't yet incorporated your respective eating plans into your lives, it's probably unrealistic to expect that either of you has lost weight. But even at this stage, some polymorphs notice an attitudinal change. Just in the process of keeping the Food Diary, for example, they have acquired some insights into when they eat and why. This information about their compulsive disorder has given them a new perspective on their overeating and, in many cases, a sense that their self-destructive eating habits can finally be changed.

So discuss with your partner how both of you are doing in relation to the program. Do you feel you've achieved some concrete accomplishments already? Have you learned something about how your relationships with people may be influencing your eating behavior?

Spend a few minutes now discussing these issues or anything else on your mind today.

FOOD DIARY

For nearly the entire remainder of today's meeting, you and your partner will share with one another your completed Food Diaries. Look them over together and discuss them. You'll find that you're using food in ways you were never aware of. You can expect to share such thoughts as "Look at this! Look what I did!"

Here are some of the points for the two of you to look for and discuss together:

1. *How much time do you spend eating your meals?* In Chapter 3, I discussed the appestat—the nerve center in your brain that controls your feelings of hunger but does not react to sensations of satiety or fullness until about twenty minutes after food is consumed. So if you eat quickly, you will have probably swallowed more food—and calories—than your body needs by the time the satiation message reaches the brain.

Many polymorphs learn to eat more slowly by using a behavior-modification technique in which they chew every bite slowly and carefully. Between bites, they put their fork down deliberately, not lifting it again until they have swallowed everything in their mouth. You, too, can learn to make eating a relaxed experience with a little awareness and some attention to your habits.

2. *What were your moods when you ate?* As I've suggested, most polymorphs eat in response to various emotions and feelings—boredom, depression, happiness, exhaustion, contentment, sexual arousal, resentment, frustration, and so on. Try to determine which moods influence your eating the most. Do you tend to have unexpected snacks when you're tired? Or when you're under pressure? Or when you're happy? Also look at your choices of food. Do you always eat chocolate when you're feeling depressed? Are cookies or crackers a favorite indulgence in response to anger?

Once you are aware of the relationship between mood and food, you must find another, more constructive response—rather than eating—to an emotion that usually makes you eat. For instance, if you are angry, try speaking straightforwardly to the person provoking your mood; if you're tired, take a nap; if you're bored or depressed, begin a pleasurable activity. As you will discover later in this program, physical exercise or a relaxation technique can also soothe emotional unrest. Many polymorphs also discover that just the support and caring of a partner can often take the place of food during a particularly vulnerable moment.

3. *Where do you usually eat?* At the dining room table? Or over the stove? In the den? In your car? Each one of these places can be a cue or a signal for you to eat. If you regularly nibble when you are in the car or while sitting at your office desk, you may be eating there unconsciously, habitually, even when you are not hungry. Also, you're less aware of *how much* you're eating if you eat on the run, snacking here and there. As a polymorph, you should commit yourself now to eating at just one place—like the dining room table—and eat *only* there.

4. *What other activities do you engage in when you eat?* When you read, watch TV, or talk on the phone while eating, these distractions make you less conscious of the act of eating. Not only might you fail to recognize how much food you are consuming but, as is true of *where* you eat, these various activities soon become cues to eat. So, for instance, every time you turn on the TV you will look for something to munch on. Or whenever you curl up with a novel in one hand you will have learned to rrab a box of cookies with the other. To combat this problem, be aware of the associations you make between certain activities and food, and teach yourself to devote your eating time *only* to eating.

5. *Do you eat alone or with other people?* Through their diaries, some people discover that when they dine with

particular people they usually overeat. Perhaps these people create tension or anxiety that the polymorph copes with by excessive eating. If you notice that you tend to overeat with certain people, examine the Food Diary for your moods at those times. Were you anxious or angry each time you ate with those individuals? Until your compulsive overeating is under control, you should consider not dining with people who seem to cause you to overeat.

Some polymorphs learn that they overeat only when they're alone, barely eating at all in the company of others. They may be embarrassed to eat in front of others because of their obesity. Or they may find that eating is so special and intimate an activity for them that they really don't want to share it with others. Individuals like these must commit themselves to never eating alone until they have learned to control their polymorphism.

6. *Was the meal or snack prepared by you or by someone else?* Many polymorphs eat constantly while they are cooking meals or cleaning up the kitchen, supposedly tasting the food to ensure that it is being prepared properly or making sure nothing is "wasted." If your Food Diary shows that you eat frequently while cooking or cleaning up, encourage your spouse or your children to fix their own snacks and help out in the kitchen. When you're in the kitchen, don't forget your pledge to eat only at the dining room table (or whatever site you've chosen). If you feel obligated to sample the meal while it is being cooked, take a spoonful with you to the dining room, sit down, and taste it there. Make random eating as complex an ordeal as possible.

In addition to these major issues that are reflected in your Food Diary, you and your partner can evaluate your eating habits in even more depth by looking over each other's records of the last few days and discussing the following subjects:

What seem to be your favorite snack foods—the ones you seemingly eat most compulsively?

Do you become preoccupied with the thought of food during the day? Under what circumstances?

Do you eat secretly so that the people in your life won't know how much you eat?

Do you feel guilty about eating?

Do you always eat everything on your plate? Do you eat the leftovers on other people's plates?

Are you aware of being hungrier or eating more at certain times of the day?

All these issues are intended as a springboard for a conversation with your partner about what you eat, the circumstances surrounding your eating, and your general attitudes toward food. As you and your partner examine each other's Food Diaries, you will each see patterns that the other doesn't. Each of us has a subconscious defense system that is operating all the time, keeping us from consciously perceiving our own destructive eating behaviors. These defenses are one reason why you've never been able to lose weight permanently in the past. Your own defenses are designed to work only for you, not someone else, and thus they are more obvious to others than they are to you. With this no-diet program, your partner can help you see through your defenses, just as you will see through his. While you might prefer to talk about the least-threatening areas, he can guide you into exploring the most significant ones. You can function in a very therapeutic way for one another by exchanging diaries and discussing them.

During your dialogue, I'd like you each to ask one another whether you left something off the diary. Perhaps there was a cookie or a candy bar that you couldn't resist but were embarrassed to record on the chart. Or how about a bite of cake that "hardly amounted to anything"? In my experience, *everyone* leaves something out of the diary. By making a note of it now, elevating it into conscious awareness, you can finally set about changing such self-defeating behavior.

As you and your partner continue talking about the diary and your attitudes toward food, keep in mind that neither of you will benefit from being critical or judgmental. Your purpose is to point out tendencies in your friend's eating. Mention them, but don't judge them. One polymorph realized that she was asking the wrong questions in relation to her partner's moods while snacking: "At first I asked her, 'What's all this anxiety you have?' But I realized how judgmental that was. The next time, I said, 'It seems like there's a lot of anxiety, and you eat when there's anxiety. *I guess I do that, too.* I notice we both do.'" The latter statement was nonthreatening, and so her partner felt comfortable responding to it. She felt free to explore the issue of her anxiety thoroughly in a safe, friendly environment.

Another polymorph recalled that her partner said, "I just closed down a Jack-in-the-Box by eating up their inventory." She laughed at the statement and then responded, "Oh, tell me about it." She didn't criticize—"You did *what?* What a crazy thing to do! You should never do that!" Avoid sitting in judgment of your partner and using words like "should" and "ought." If you are supportive of one another, you will both gradually start understanding your compulsive overeating.

One woman told me that her diary helped her realize how unhappy eating made her. "While I was eating and afterward, I didn't feel good about what was going on," she recalled. "I never recognized that before. I thought I was eating to make me feel good, but it wasn't working." Another polymorph realized that she binged whenever she was depressed. "Instead of crying like other people do, I'd go to the refrigerator," she explained. "It didn't make any sense, but I never understood what was going on until my partner and I studied my diary closely."

In the next few days, you will notice the impact that this discussion of your Food Diary has had on your life. When you're angry, for example, and reach for some food, you will be more aware of it than you've ever been before. You've discussed it in a nonthreatening atmosphere, and there will have already been some unconscious changes in behavior that will aid you in abstaining from that food. The insights arrived at by you and your partner will help set you on the proper course toward permanent weight control.

In the days between now and your next meeting, continue keeping the Food Diary. Once again, don't try to consciously change *what* you eat, but this time, feel free to try changing *how* and *why* you eat—for instance, by dining in a specific place, eliminating all associated activities, trying to eat more slowly, being aware of your moods, etc. Use the Food Diary to maintain an accurate record of your eating experiences.

PREPARING FOR THE TASTING EXERCISE

Before this session with your partner ends, plan together an exercise that you will do at the next meeting. At that time, you each should have on hand small portions of five food items of various textures and tastes: (1) a *sweet* food; (2) a *sour* one; (3) a *chewy* or *crunchy* one; (4) a *smooth* one; and (5) a *juicy* one. Also provide a blindfold or a handkerchief that can be used to cover your eyes during the experience. This exercise is intended to make you more sensitive to the tastes and textures of food than you've ever been before. So make a commitment to each other that you will each have these items at the next meeting.

DAY 2

EVALUATING YOUR PROGRESS

Spend the first few minutes of today's session examining and discussing with your partner any thoughts you are having relative to this program. For instance, are you feeling some accomplishment? Do you sense any personal frustration or resistance? Has your behavior undergone any changes as a result of the discussions you've already had? Talk to your partner openly about whatever is on your mind. Reaffirm to each other your commitment to this ten-week regimen.

Today you will be introduced to the food plan with its built-in support system (the calling-in plan) and the physical exercise program—two critically important elements in this book. After this meeting, you will be well into the overall program and will begin noticing significant progress from week to week.

Take a few minutes now to examine one another's Food Diaries, which you have kept over the last few days. Follow the same guidelines as at the last meeting, examining how your mood and other factors have influenced your eating behavior. In just the past couple of days, by adhering to the techniques discussed last time, you probably experienced some meaningful changes. Share your feelings about these early improvements in your eating habits. Continue keeping the Food Diary for the days between now and your next meeting.

THE CALLING-IN PLAN

You and your partner will each start following your special food plans tomorrow. You will begin a sensible eating program that will not deprive you emotionally, physically, or nutritionally. Although you won't be on a diet, the foods you choose are significant, and we will discuss them in a moment. But just as important is the support system that will be built into the plan. It will involve a daily telephone call to your partner, probably in the morning, reporting on all the food you are planning to eat that day. In essence, you will decide in advance what you are going to eat and simply tell your partner about it.

There are several purposes for this calling-in system, and I want you and your partner to become familiar with them now. First, like the Food Diary, it will bring your respective eating behaviors into conscious awareness. Not only will you have the diary to remind you of what you are eating, but you will also now be verbalizing your menu to your partner. During the day, if you decide to alter your diet in any way, you must give your partner a call *beforehand* and tell him. Simply report, "We're having guests tonight, and dessert will be chocolate cake. I'm planning to have a slice with everyone else." You must make every attempt to contact your partner, no matter what time of the day or night. If you are unable to reach him, *you* must write down the change and report it to him the next time the two of you talk.

The calling-in system will require both of you to make commitments about your choices of food and take responsibility for what you eat. If you impulsively feel like making yourself an ice cream sundae, there is a strong deterrent against doing so if you have to call your partner first to report your intentions. Most polymorphs in this program find it easier *not* to binge than to call their partner and announce that they are going to.

If either you or your partner is already feeling some resistance to a daily telephone report of your menu, you should discuss it now. Perhaps you find the concept too time-consuming (it's not; it only requires about three minutes a day). Maybe you think it's going to be an annoying thing to do, day after day. Perhaps you feel uncomfortable about verbally reporting *everything* you eat—from an extra carrot stick to a banana split.

As uneasy as the concept may make you feel now, this approach has proven extremely successful in treating many kinds of compulsive disorders, including overeating. Organizations like Overeaters Anonymous use a similar technique to help thousands of members. Studies indicate that the most significant elements at work here are the psychological and emotional benefits from the support that your partner may be able to offer you in a time of "crisis."

If you feel like bingeing—if you feel like you absolutely *must* have a piece of cake that is not on your daily food plan—you can discuss this compulsive feeling with your partner. He can offer you some priceless and helpful qualities, including his warmth, compassion, understanding, and common sense. If you are depressed and think only food can make you feel better, tell your partner. He can help you sort out your thoughts so that you can decide whether a piece of cake is really the answer to your anxieties.

As with all the other components of this program, your partner is there to hear the information, not to pass judgment. If you report, "I'm going to have a hot fudge sundae for a snack at 3:00 P.M.," he might ask, "Would you like to discuss this?" But he should *not* try to dissuade you, no matter how gently, from eating the sundae. His function is to serve as a mirror, to help you comprehend your intended behavior and your anxieties clearly. It may be heard to keep from saying, "You were doing so well . . . why do you want to ruin it with a hot fudge sundae?" But he mustn't.

One of the most common problems of the polymorph is that other people take responsibility for his overeating. Someone else worries about it, advises and/or pesters him about it, and tries to regulate it. He never learns how to control his eating behavior himself, and any related feelings of poor self-esteem he may have are never dealt with on any meaningful level.

For you to lose weight permanently, *you* are going to have to take responsibility for your behavior and make the changes happen. So it makes no sense for your partner to be judgmental. That is what everyone has done to you for years. It hasn't worked in the past, and it will never work. Your partner's job is simply to restate what he hears, to reflect back everything you're doing, and make certain that you are aware of your own thoughts and feelings and the reasons behind them. You, of course, should do the same for him. Once you really start seeing yourself, and recognizing and understanding your behavior, then *you* can begin to take control of the situation. Eventually, *you* will decide not to eat that hot fudge sundae if it is not in your best interest to do so.

So during today's meeting, set up a time when you and your partner will talk each day (right before breakfast works best for many people). During your three-minute daily conversation, you will read one another your respective menus, which you have written out in advance. Make the call in a quiet place where you won't be interrupted. Even if your food plan is the same as it was the day before, you must call it in to your partner *every* day. As you hear it over the phone, each of you will write down the other's eating plan. It is no more complicated than that.

YOUR NO-DIET FOOD PLAN

Having established the ground rules for calling in, it's now time for you and your partner to decide upon your personal eating plans. There are some specific food programs that I consider worthwhile, but none of them is a "magic diet." The only way to lose weight, regardless of *what* you eat, is to expend more caloric units than you take in. And there is no point in consuming grapes, grapefruits, protein, or whatever else happens to be in vogue just to lose five or ten pounds if you are only going to gain it back as soon as you return to your old eating patterns.

I could even offer you my own miracle diet—the "Rader Magic Diet." Every time you feel like eating, it requires that you go to a closet, step inside, close the door, and stay there until you don't feel like eating anymore. I guarantee you'll lose weight with it, but I also guarantee you'll gain it all back—and more. "Get-thin-quick" schemes are just as unrealistic as most "get-rich-quick" contrivances.

So we all know how to lose weight; keeping it off is the polymorph's problem. And you won't be able to accomplish permanent weight loss until you have made some significant changes in your life. To help you lose your excess weight and maintain that weight loss for good, a sound nutritional program is essential, one in which you learn to eat sensibly and nutritionally while maintaining your health.

By eating "sensibly," I simply mean adopting a food plan that supplies the basics of good nutrition—proteins, carbohydrates, and fats. As a general guideline, if you do not exercise much, you should eat ten calories per day for each pound you weigh to *maintain* your current weight; consuming fewer than ten would cause weight *loss*. If you are physically active, eating fourteen calories per day for each pound you weigh would *maintain* your current weight; consuming fewer than fourteen would result in weight reduction. Thus, if you weigh 135 pounds and are generally inactive, you must consume fewer than 1350 calories (135 × 10) a day to lose weight.

In the appendix of this book I have provided a choice of several food plans. They've been tested by and proven successful for literally thousands of people. If you follow them, you *will* achieve and maintain permanent weight loss.

If you prefer, feel free to choose an eating program of your own—perhaps one that has helped you lose weight in the past—as long as it's nutritionally well balanced. Any diet that eliminates important, basic foods (milk, vegetables, breads, cereals, etc.) can lead to serious nutritional deficiencies and metabolic imbalances. If you don't avoid these kinds of diets, you will not only risk illness, but also find yourself craving "forbidden foods" and making matters worse by bingeing.

If you have been on (and off) diets for years, you probably know exactly what I mean by a food plan that is "nutritionally sound." Most overweight people, after all, are "experts" on food and nutrition. But, as general guidelines, any eating plan you adopt should possess the following characteristics.

1. A variety of high-valued vegetable and animal protein. These should be obtained from lean meat, fish, shellfish, poultry, eggs, and milk products. Peas, nuts, beans, and soybeans also are good protein sources.

2. A minimum level of fats. Fats are essential in moderate amounts for your body to function properly. But too many fats can increase your risk of coronary heart disease and add too many calories to your food plan (fat provides more than twice the calories per gram than protein and carbohydrates do). I suggest that you obtain fats from foods with relatively low levels of fat—lamb chops, lean ground beef, pot roast, broiled fish and chicken, and cottage cheese—while avoiding such high-fat foodstuffs as butter, margarine, mayonnaise, and walnuts.

3. A variety of carbohydrate sources—fruits, vegetables, whole grains, and legumes.

4. Adequate amounts of vitamins and minerals, which can be obtained naturally in many fresh foods, including leafy green or yellow vegetables, potatoes, lean meat, citrus fruits and juices, eggs, nuts, and legumes.

5. A minimal amount of refined sugar. You will probably never be able to eliminate sugar from your diet completely (it is a hidden ingredient in many prepared foods). But take steps to reduce your sugar intake, perhaps by eating fresh (rather than

canned) fruits or by not putting sugar in your coffee or on your cereal (sweeten it with strawberries or raisins instead). Also, read food labels and avoid foods with sugar listed high among their ingredients.

6. Sufficient amounts of fiber. We all need fiber to help our digestive systems operate properly. You will obtain all the fiber you need by eating everyday foods like beans, cabbage, carrots, fruits, parsnips, and artichokes.

7. Daily sensible portions of each of the four basic food groups:

Dairy: nonfat milk, yogurt.

Fruits and vegetables: cabbage, cauliflower, celery, broccoli, lettuce, spinach, oranges, grapefruits, apples.

Breads and cereals: rice, dried beans, cereals, whole-grain bread.

Meats and proteins: poultry, fish, cottage cheese, meat.

It is essential for you and your partner to commit yourselves today to a food program that will allow you to lose weight gradually and keep it off. Talk with your partner about eating programs that you think will work for you, and carefully review those in the appendix. Whatever plan you choose, it will become *yours*. This is the one you will be calling in to your partner every day, deviating from it *only* after telling your partner you intend to do so.

TALKING ABOUT WITHDRAWAL

You and your partner may both experience some uncomfortable times during the first few days of your new eating plans. As levels of sugar are reduced in your diet, you might experience withdrawal symptoms not unlike those of an addict to any other drug. As I discussed in Chapter 3, you may feel anxious, tense, irritable, fidgety, disoriented, or tearful. There is both a physiological and a psychological component to this withdrawal phenomenon, as both your body and your mind adjust to the absence of this chemical. It's all part of the process, but at least now you will know why it is happening. When you experience these unpleasant symptoms, you will feel a craving for food. Instead, reach out for your partner.

"I was feeling terrrible on the fourth night of my eating plan," recalled Lana. "I was so stressed. I phoned my partner and told her that I had just snapped at my husband, and that I felt like I was out of control. She listened, and then reminded me, 'Dr. Rader said this would happen. It's okay to be irritable. Tell your husband that you're going to be a little crazy for the next few days.'" Just this reassurance soothed Lana. She could even laugh at herself afterward for her irritability.

Fortunately, these symptoms usually end after about a week. Make a commitment now with your partner that you will bear with each other if either of you experiences these symptoms, and make a telephone call instead of rushing to the refrigerator.

THE TASTING EXERCISE

In the final few minutes of this session, I would like you and your partner to perform the tasting exercise that you agreed to prepare for at the last meeting. The primary purpose of this activity is to further bring your relationship with food into conscious awareness. And when you have to concentrate on nothing but food, you may be surprised by your reaction.

1. Sit facing one another, knees almost touching, with your plates of various food items—sweet, sour, chewy, smooth,

juicy—on your laps. Take a close, last look at your plate and at your partner's, and then place the handkerchiefs or blindfolds over your eyes. Do not remove them until the exercise is completed. The idea is to concentrate on the sensations of taste and texture without sight as a distraction.

2. Pick up the sweet food and place it in *each other's* mouths. Let your partner feed you. Be aware of how you feel when someone else places food in your mouth. Remember this feeling; it will be a good discussion topic later.

3. With this sweet item in your mouth, slowly—very slowly—begin to chew it. With each bite, soak every ounce of taste out of it. Savor it. Smack your lips. As the item crumbles into tinier fragments, swirl it through your entire mouth. Take a few moments to really acquaint yourself with this food. Be as aware as possible of its taste and texture. Do not talk to your partner; concentrate solely on the food. After a minute or two, swallow.

4. Next, take the sour food from your plates and feed it to one another. Once again, go through the same process of chewing and experiencing. Become fully sensitive to the sensations in your mouth.

5. Move on to the other items on your plate, one at a time, and repeat the process. After you've progressed through them all, remove your blindfolds.

6. Now, discuss your reactions with your partner. Many people tell me that they found it very uncomfortable to be fed by their partners; some even felt nauseated. For them, the eating process—perhaps the only component of their lives that they believed was really theirs—was suddenly being manipulated from without. They had to trust another person in the outside world, and that was hard for them to do.

Most polymorphs are surprised by their responses to this exercise. "The first thing I realized," said Stanley, "was that, until this exercise, I never really tasted my food. When I eat, I gobble it down. I shove as much into my mouth as quickly as possible. I always thought I liked certain foods, but I finally had to acknowledge that I wasn't thinking about what I was doing; I wasn't even enjoying the experience. I see now that it was *eating* I liked; I never actually tasted the food."

Another polymorph said, "I just didn't get as much out of the food as I thought I would. I usually find eating a pleasant experience, but I guess I really just like the feeling of a full stomach. My partner told me that, for her, stuffing herself was sometimes a way of comforting herself and making her feel like she was loving herself from the inside. That might be what it was for me, too."

For many polymorphs, food has become a substitute for nurturing. When you feel emotionally empty inside, lonely, frustrated, and unloved, you may be trying to fill up that vacuum with food. But, in truth, only *people* can satisfy this basic human need.

Discuss this exercise with your partner. As the two of you come to recognize this pattern and become more relaxed and open with one another, you will soon find that human contact can fill you up more fully than food ever has.

FILLING OTHER NEEDS: YOUR PHYSICAL EXERCISE PROGRAM

Like food itself, exercise is a basic bodily need, and if the body is not physically challenged, it will deteriorate. But few Americans, whether they be polymorphs or not, exercise as much as they should. They exert little physical energy throughout the day. And at night they find it easier to sit in front of the TV with a dish of ice cream than to take a brisk evening walk.

If you are consistently inactive, your body is paying the price. Not only do you weigh more than you'd like to, but your body is also a good deal less efficient than it should be, operating at between 25 and 30 percent of its potential. As a polymorph, *it is absolutely essential for you to exercise regularly to maintain good physical and psychological health.* A daily exercise program can:

Burn up calories and help you lose weight faster.

Tighten flabby muscles.

Strengthen important bodily organs, including the heart, helping you live longer.

Reduce aches, pains, and stiffness.

Improve your posture.

Delay and reduce fatigue.

Improve your mood.

Help you sleep better.

The psychological advantages of exercise are just as important to the polymorph as the physical ones. Many overweight people hate their bodies and see them as enemies, as roadblocks to happiness. Their long-standing sense of inadequacy is reinforced by feelings of flaccidity and physical weakness. Exercise allows them to start taking pleasure in their bodies and, just as important, gain a sense of control over themselves. As their self-confidence and self-esteem increase, they often want to eat less. Instead of relinquishing control of their lives, exercise puts them back in command and, in doing so, dramatically changes the way they view themselves.

Beginning at your next meeting, start experiencing the physical and psychological pleasures of exercise. For fifteen minutes of that session, and during every meeting thereafter, perform some exercises designed to maximize your good health and put you back in touch with your body. By exercising together, you and your partner can reduce the boredom that many people find in exercising. You can keep each other company as well as encourage and motivate one another. Also, even during your nonmeeting days, continue to exercise regularly on your own—walking, jogging, swimming, bicycling, calisthenics. Physical activity must become a part of your daily life.

You may already have an idea of the type of exercises you would like to participate in. But if you want some guidance, I will provide you with a specific exercise plan next week. It is a program that many polymorphs have found helpful. But no matter what you eventually choose, it need not be elaborate or sophisticated. The best exercise is the kind that stimulates your cardiovascular activity, raising your heartbeat to 70 to 80 percent of its full capacity. (To determine your heart's capacity, subtract your age from 220.) That is why many polymorphs on this program choose activities like taking brisk walks or jogging.

So come to the next meeting prepared to spend a few minutes exercising. The important thing is to get your body moving and feel good about doing so.

PLANNING FOR THE NEXT MEETING

At your first meeting with your partner next week, one of you will need to provide a large paper bag and have a full-length mirror and a hand-held mirror available. As peculiar as this may sound, these are tools you will use in an exercise to help you see yourself as you really are, to allow you to grasp other elements of your polymorphism. It would be helpful to wear tight-fitting clothes to that meeting, which reveal your shape more than you might like. Also, bring a change of clothes to wear when you and your partner exercise.

Week 3

DAY 1

EVALUATING YOUR PROGRESS

You and your partner should have a lot to talk about today. Since your last meeting, the two of you have not only been continuing your Food Diaries, but you have also adopted your eating plans and started the calling-in system. In the first part of today's meeting, focus your discussion on these important facets of the program.

The calling-in system and the eating plan are good starting points. You and your partner may have had more difficulty with them than you might have presumed, even with all your good intentions. This sensible new eating plan is often a dramatic departure from the polymorph's normal food habits. Negative eating behavior that has taken years to develop can't be changed overnight. Spend some time evaluating your experiences over the last few days.

The questions below might help you open your discussion:

Did you keep to the eating plan that you had created for yourself? Were there any difficulties in doing so?

Did you frequently want to alter your diet? If so, what are some of the reasons you wished to do so?

How often did you actually make changes? Just once or several times a day? What was going on in your life at these times?

Did you ever "cheat" by not calling your partner when you made a change? How can you make yourself more conscientious about calling in the future?

Was there ever a time when you didn't call your partner for one of your daily prearranged telephone sessions? If so, why?

Do you anticipate that things will get easier in the upcoming weeks? Or do you foresee problems?

Carmen recalls a problem that she had on the third day of the calling-in plan. "I ate a bite of a friend's doughnut during our coffee break at work without calling my partner in advance. And I felt so guilty that I decided never to tell my partner about it. That's where my real trouble started. I became very anxious about this deception, and that night I found myself bingeing. Then I finally called my partner and explained everything. She was very supportive, and I felt that a huge burden had been lifted from my shoulders. It was an experience that brought me and my partner closer."

If either you or your partner has had a problem, just recommit yourself to making this program work. Plan now for your next telephone conversation. Discuss any major modifications either of you wants to make in your regular diet. Perhaps your doctor has given you a well-balanced eating plan that you are thinking about adopting. Or perhaps you have seen a diet in a magazine that sounds appealing. If you'd like to begin one of these plans, do so now. But make certain that it's one that you can stick with and that it's carefully balanced.

Many times in the upcoming weeks, after you have made your daily call to your partner, you will probably think of a dozen excuses for deviating from the menu that you have reported. One woman told me, "I cooked some fish for dinner, but it tasted terrible, so I raided the cookie jar and ate some cookies instead." A man said, "The grocery store closed early on Sunday and I couldn't buy the right foods, so I had to substitute." A woman rationalized, "I didn't want to make my aunt feel self-conscious that she was the only one eating the mashed potatoes, so I joined her." Be honest with yourself, and try to keep these deviations to a minimum. When they do happen, your partner must be told about them *before* you substitute for this program to be effective.

One polymorph consistently told her partner, "I was going to call to tell you about the food I added to my plan, but I didn't want to bother you at work." More than likely, she was experiencing what Carmen did—guilt and embarrassment. But there's nothing to be embarrassed about. Your partner won't judge or scold you. Instead, his job is to be accepting of what you're going through and supportive if you need support. After all, he is probably experiencing the same things.

Once you finally settle in with a food program, even if it takes you a while to find one that works for you, this will be the one you will stay with. Approach it one day at a time rather than thinking about the weeks still ahead of you. Concentrate only on today. In doing so, sensible eating habits will gradually become part of your life.

After the discussion of the calling-in and food plans, spend a few minutes reviewing your Food Diary with your partner. If you wavered from your prearranged eating schedule in the last few days, try to discover the reasons why by studying the chart carefully. Do you seem to snack uncontrollably when you're bored? Or when you're depressed? Or happy? In the future, whenever you sense yourself in one of these binge-provoking moods, call your partner for support rather than submitting to the temptation of food, and make these calls in private since family members may misunderstand some of the things you're saying. Continue keeping the Food

Diary for a few more days. It's providing you with significant information about your behavior.

This is also the time to discuss any other problems or issues that may be relevant to your life or this program. Some polymorphs are still timid about really opening up with their partner at this stage. If you are having this problem, talk it over with your friend. The mere act of discussing your anxiety can usually diminish it, particularly if your partner acknowledges that he too has some tension.

THE PAPER-BAG EXERCISE

The paper-bag exercise will yield some important information for this no-diet program. Before you and your partner begin it, let me explain its basis.

Over the years, we have all created mental images of the way we see our bodies. And as I discussed in Chapter 2, polymorphs often create denial systems that manufacture *false* images of who they are, and thus their perceptions of themselves are often distorted. For this reason, many compulsive overeaters do not know what their bodies really look like. They have chosen to shield themselves from the problem by attempting to deceive themselves about their weight. They wear loose-fitting clothes that don't emphasize their more obvious bulges and which, in a real sense, have become their disguises. Ironically, the public is so accustomed to associating loose-fitting clothes with obesity that even a thin person wearing these clothes is often thought to be overweight. And the distorted body image that they have created for themselves prevents them from ever realistically facing up to the weight-loss task ahead of them.

For you and your partner to succeed in this program, you must understand the differences between how you perceive yourself and how you really look. You must gain an insight into some of the self-deceptions you have engaged in. This exercise will help you accomplish that.

You and your partner will cut eyeholes in the paper bag you have brought with you, and then each will take a turn putting the bag over your head, looking into a full-length mirror, and describing aloud what you see. With your face covered, you will be forced to really look at the rest of yourself, perhaps for the first time in years, observing and evaluating your body objectively, as if it belonged to someone else.

You need not be naked for this exercise to be effective. If you have worn tight-fitting clothes that reveal your shape rather than disguise it, this experience will be very worthwhile.

So let's get started, with either you or your partner placing the bag over your head and standing in front of a full-length mirror. Spend a minute or two just examining yourself from neck to toe, really concentrating on what is in front of you. Then turn around and, using the hand mirror as well, concentrate on the back view.

What do you see? Begin telling your partner aloud how you look to yourself, but refer to your body in the third person, as if it belonged to someone else. What do you like? What don't you like? Note the descriptive words and phrases you use. Of course, it will be hard not to be subjective and opinionated, but try to be absolutely frank and unbiased about what you see.

Your partner's role during this exercise is to guide you. "Let's isolate the parts of the body. . . . What do you think of his/her arms? . . . What do you think of his/her legs?" Continue through the rest of the body. As your partner serves as your guide, he will listen to your responses, but should not be judgmental about them.

Once you have had the chance to perform this exercise, your partner will take a turn. Guide him in the same way that he helped you. Listen, but don't prompt, judge, or console. Just let him tell you what he sees.

After each of you has experienced this exercise, discuss it with one another. But now talk about what you saw in the first person. How did *you* feel? Sad? Anxious? Angry? Depressed? Worried? Content? Neutral? What surprises did you encounter? Were you shocked by how successfully you have ignored your body in the past? Did some parts of your anatomy look worse than the body image you might have created for yourself? Did some parts look better?

This exercise typically opens up many avenues of discussion. Many polymorphs may feel threatened by this exercise. Their bodies are strangers to them and, after taking a hard look, they may not like what they see. If that's what you're feeling, share it with your partner.

One polymorph told me, "I was in a lot of stress during this exercise, and I'm thankful that my partner was there to help me deal with it. But as we talked, we both realized that there was also a great relief of anxiety. We had finally faced up to our overweight, and knew that we didn't want to spend the rest of our lives fooling ourselves about it."

The paper-bag exercise also helps most polymorphs better understand their self-esteem. In study after study, psychiatrists and psychologists have discovered the strong relationship between a negative body image and poor self-esteem. The way you feel about yourself, and the way you face life each day, is determined in great part by the way you perceive your physical being. And, for most polymorphs, that self-image is lower than it could be, as this exercise will demonstrate.

Fortunately, you and your partner can learn to successfully control your overeating compulsion. But it is going to take more than an eating plan and an exercise program to improve your self-esteem, even though these are essential parts of the process. You will also need to begin to deal with some of the issues, such as how you feel others perceive you, as described in this ten-week, no-diet plan. Although approaches like the paper-bag exercise may seem simplistic on the surface, my experience is that they can help open up discussion on significant areas related to negative self-esteem.

EXERCISING

Exercise is a well-documented method for improving your physical appearance, your personal body image, and your self-esteem. As you feel better, you'll progressively look better to yourself in a continuous cycle.

At your last meeting, you and your partner agreed to participate in fifteen minutes of exercise a day. So during today's meeting, preferably at or near the beginning, be sure to actively start your physical-fitness program. Change into your exercising clothes and get started.

The two of you may use an exercise plan of your own choosing, but if neither of you has brought one along today, follow the carefully conceived fitness routine below. It consists of eight exercises, which you both should do together, with only short pauses between each one. They have been selected specifically for the polymorph, with three primary objectives in mind: (1) increased flexibility, (2) muscle toning, and (3) cardiovascular conditioning. They are not new or revolutionary exercises, but are time-tested calisthenics that have been incorporated into many highly respected fitness regimens, including those at West Point and the Royal Canadian Air Force. Don't feel that you have to do each one perfectly or at a rapid pace, particularly in the beginning. But eventually, the faster you can move through them, the more rapid your heart will beat, and the more benefit you'll derive from them. Let's begin.

1. Trunk Bend. This is an excellent stretching exercise for the entire tody. Stand erect with your feet comfortably apart and your arms extended above your head. Bend at the waist and try to touch the floor just to the right of your right foot. (Just bend as far as feels comfortable to you.) Retreat slightly, and then try directly touching your toes. Retreat slightly again, and try touching the floor just to the left of the left foot. Then return to the upright position and repeat the routine. Try ten repetitions, or as many as you feel comfortable doing.

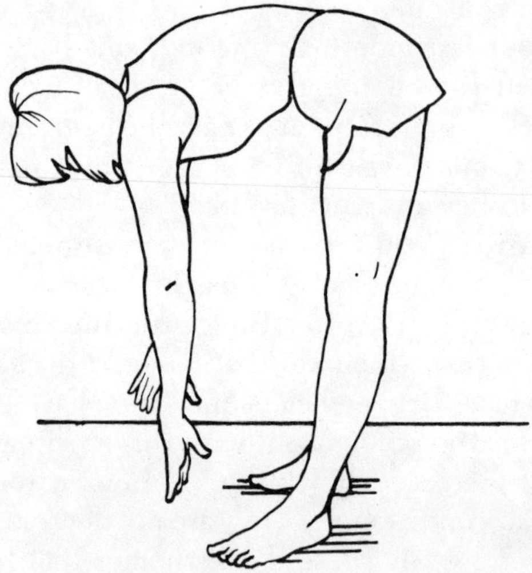

2. Body Bender. This exercise is designed to work on your waist. Stand erect, with your feet comfortably apart and your hands interlaced behind your neck. Bend your trunk sideward to the left as far as you can, keeping your hands behind your neck. Return to the upright position and then bend to the right. Try ten repetitions to the left and ten to the right.

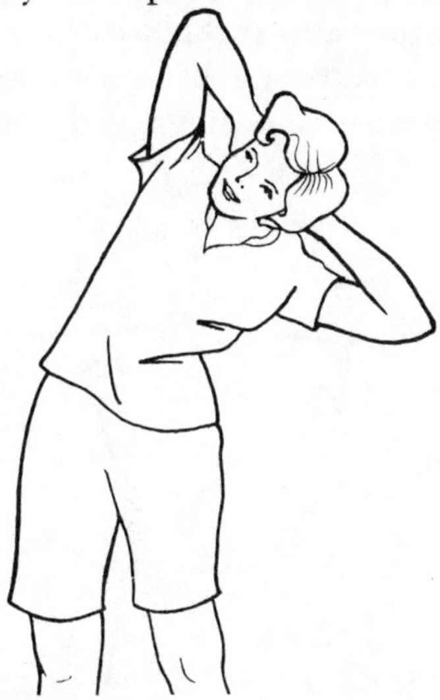

3. Floor Bender. This is an excellent exercise for the hips. Lie on your back, eyes to the ceiling, with your arms extended out to the sides, palms down on the floor. Bring your knees up toward the chest and then, with both your knees and ankles touching, roll your knees to the left side, letting them touch the floor. Then raise them and lower them to the right side. Repeat ten times on each side if possible.

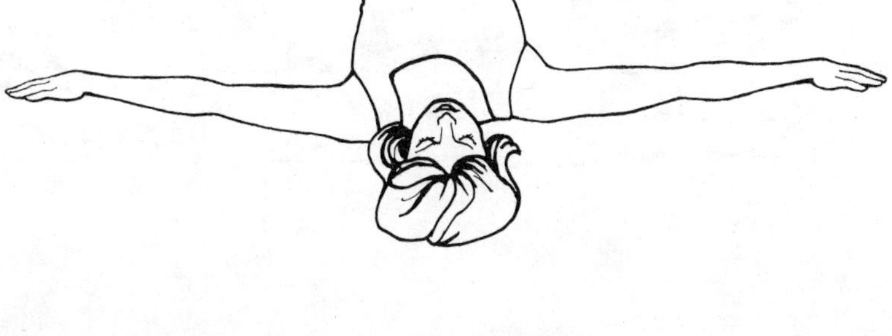

4. *Arm Circles.* This exercise will work on the shoulders, chest, upper back, and arms. Stand erect and extend your arms outward to the sides at shoulder height, with your palms facing up. Then, with your eyes looking straight ahead, rotate your arms clockwise ten times and counterclockwise ten times.

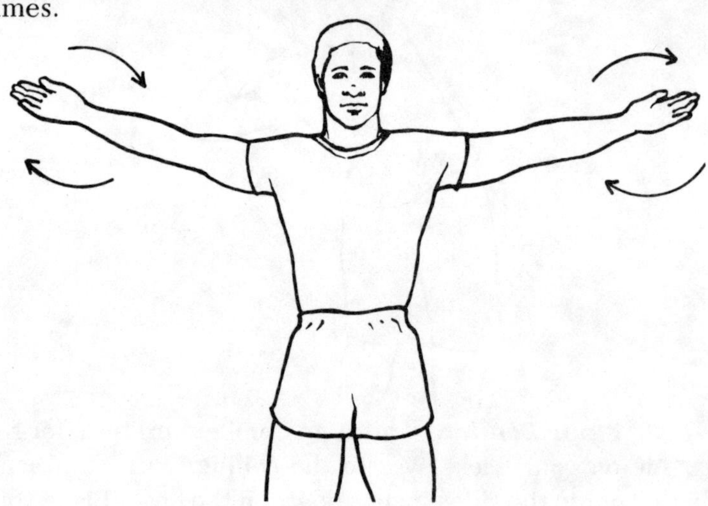

5. *Head Curls.* Your abdomen and the front of your thighs will benefit from this exercise. Lie on your back, with your arms at your sides, palms down. As you tighten your stomach muscles, lift your head, shoulders, and elbows slightly off the floor. Keep them elevated for three seconds and then return to the starting position. Repeat five times.

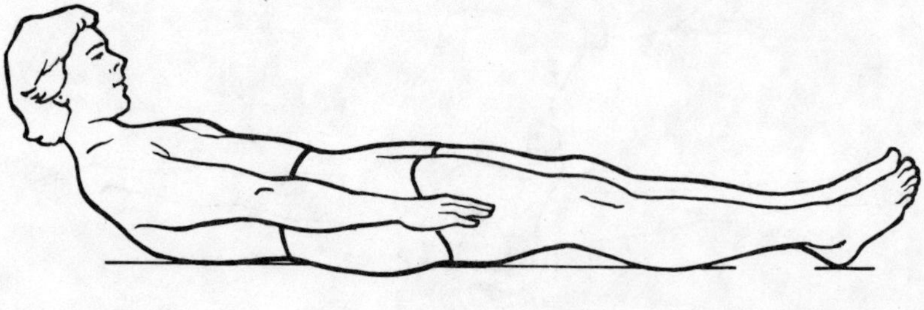

6. Knee Lifts. This exercise will work on your lower back and hips. Stand erect, with your feet comfortably apart and your arms by your sides. Raise your right knee as high as possible and then, while keeping your back straight, grasp your leg with both hands and pull your knee toward your body. Lower the right knee and repeat with the left. Try ten repetitions with the left and ten with the right.

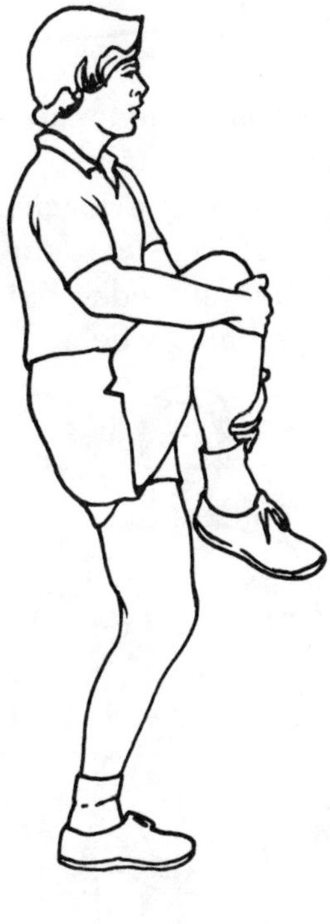

7. Leg Lifts. This exercise is designed to benefit primarily the sides of your thighs. Lie on your right side, propping your head on your right hand, with your left hand braced on the floor for support. Keeping your left leg straight, raise it as high as possible, and then lower it. Repeat ten times, and then switch sides, raising the right leg ten times.

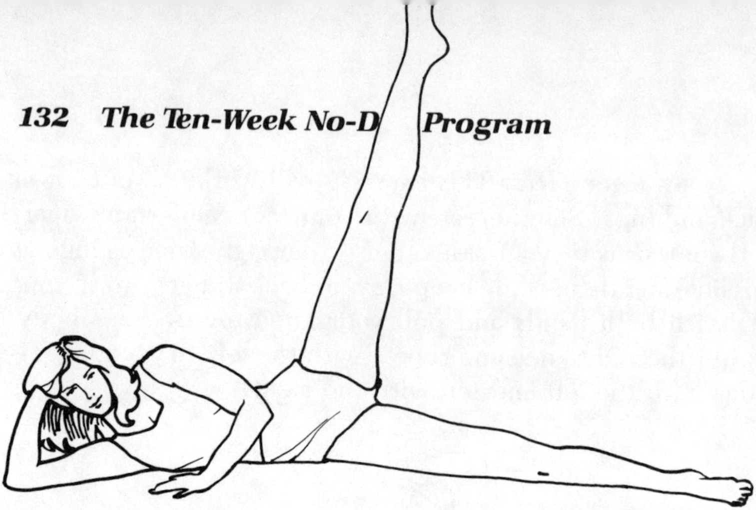

8. Running in Place. Your cardiovascular system will be challenged in this exercise. Stand in a relaxed position with your arms at your sides. Begin jogging up and down at a comfortable pace, raising your feet four to six inches off the floor. Continue for one minute today, but gradually build up to four minutes in the upcoming weeks.

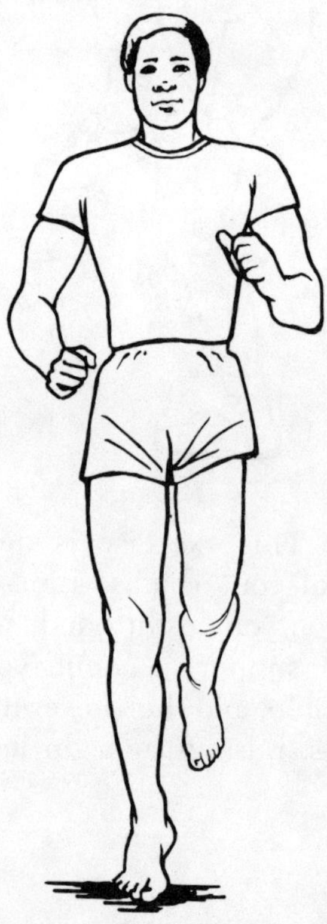

As you begin these exercises, don't be concerned if you can't do much more than go through the motions. Exercising will gradually become easier as you grow more accustomed to it. A few weeks from now, as your endurance increases, you'll tire less quickly, not only while performing these exercises, but also while carrying out your daily activities. And you'll also be happily surprised at how regular exercise can improve your mood.

It is a common group-therapy technique to start sessions with some physical exercise to relax and loosen up the participants. Permit yourself to feel good about your physical self, and you'll start loosening the grip that polymorphism has had upon you for years.

DAY 2

EVALUATING YOUR PROGRESS

During this meeting, discuss with your partner once again the progress you are making in this program. The two of you are now approaching the end of the third week, and you may already be noticing some dramatic improvements in yourself. Many polymorphs report that they already feel that they may have lost a few pounds. They are also optimistic about significantly changing many other aspects of their life in this ten-week program. An approach like this one, which explores and deals with such issues as self-esteem and interpersonal relationships, cannot help but eventually affect every component of your life while teaching you to permanently manage your compulsive overeating.

In today's discussion with your partner, review the progress and problems you are experiencing in relation to the biweekly meetings, the food plan, the daily call-ins, the Food

Diary, and the exercise program. Is it becoming easier to adhere to your food plan, or are you still deviating from it frequently? Are you less hesitant about phoning your partner to report a change, or are you still embarrassed to do so? Does your Food Diary reflect that you are learning *how* to eat—chewing slowly, eliminating associated activities, and avoiding people and situations that may stimulate bingeing? Do you feel any resistance to attending these twice-a-week meetings, or do you genuinely look forward to them now?

At one time or another, everyone experiences periods of regression—backsliding or bingeing—so don't be upset when they happen to you. During this week, for example, because you have changed your eating habits and are probably consuming less sugar, you may be feeling some of the withdrawal symptoms I have told you about. For years, you have been, in a sense, a sugar "addict," and as you reduce your intake of this "drug" your body and mind may respond with temporary headaches, dizziness, nervousness, and irritability. During these times, you may have felt the urge to reach for sugar or sweetened foods to ease these uncomfortable symptoms.

When either of you slips from the eating plan, reaching for unscheduled foods, be especially supportive of one another. With each other's encouragement, you will pass through these periods relatively quickly. Renew your commitment to stick it out.

SIZING UP YOUR SELF-ESTEEM

The paper-bag exercise at the last meeting may have been both anxiety-producing and extremely helpful. For the first time in years, you may have taken a true look at your body.

We all want to be liked, not only by the people around us, but also by ourselves. But for most people—whether they are fat or thin, smart or slow, outgoing or introverted—there is an inward negative judgment they make on themselves. Therefore, *no man or woman feels as worthwhile as he or she truly is.*

As I discussed earlier in the book, polymorphs are often enraged at themselves for being overweight, for eating compulsively, and for having failed at countless diets. Negative impressions like these become their self-image, no matter how many positive qualities they may possess as well; bad feelings about the way they look overpowers everything else.

In this session, you and your partner will explore this issue of self-esteem. For the next thirty minutes, I want the two of you to take turns discussing how you feel about yourself. Here are some questions to help you get started:

Are you happy in your life?

Do you have as many or more positive qualities as negative ones?

Do you feel differently about yourself now than at any time when you were thinner?

Are you as worthwhile a person as the people with whom you live, work, and socialize?

Are you deserving of the love and/or friendship of the people around you?

Do you view your polymorphism as "punishment" for something you have done in your life?

Do you like yourself?

During this discussion, you will learn a lot about yourself. Here's the way the process worked for a polymorph named Michael. "I found it very disturbing to deal with this issue of self-esteem," he recalls, "and so I just told my partner how good I felt about myself, and how I couldn't figure out why some overweight people are so self-deprecating.

"My partner let me talk, nodded his head a few times, and seemed to understand. But when he started to discuss the same issues, he didn't sound anything like me. He told me how little he thought of himself in general, that he couldn't do anything right—from being a father and husband to losing weight. He was describing my own feelings exactly, but I had been afraid to say it. And I finally told him that.

"I also told him that I couldn't understand why he felt so terrible about himself. I thought he was a decent guy, a very worthy person. He said exactly the same things about me. All the negative energy in our lives seemed to be coming from within us, not from the outside world. We were so busy belittling ourselves that we never saw the good parts of us that others saw."

When polymorphs describe themselves, few of them say that they have a compulsive disease. Instead, they label themselves with words like "weak-willed" or "inadequate." You must let go of that negative self-concept. It is true that you are overweight, but by no means does that describe your whole person. Your excess pounds are only a small part of you; they hardly tell the whole story of your personality, your accomplishments, and the people who love and trust you.

As your partner talks about himself, give him your total attention. Help him define his thoughts and feelings, which will sometimes make him realize how irrationally he has been treating himself. "I was being very unfair," recalled one polymorph. "I was so angry at myself that I never saw a balanced picture—my good points as well as the bad. I was overweight, but I also had accomplished a lot in my career, and was raising two very special kids. I finally realized that I didn't have to be perfect."

Don't give advice to your partner, but let him know your feelings about him if he asks. Perhaps the greatest psychological boost he could receive today is your warmth and support.

The issue of self-esteem will be dealt with in various

forms in the upcoming weeks. With your partner's support, you will learn that you can finally start respecting and believing in yourself and, in turn, in your ability to successfully manage your polymorphism.

EXERCISING

Some time during today's meeting, preferably at or near the beginning, you and your partner should once again exercise together. I hope that in the days between your last meeting and this one you exercised at home on your own. If so, you are probably already working out the sore muscles that seem inevitable whenever a new physical-fitness program begins. Once the kinks are gone, you'll really start enjoying the sensations of your own bodily movements. And the psychological benefits—including feelings of increased vigor and energy—will be as gratifying as the physiological ones.

Keep in mind that your exercise program should be approached slowly and easily during these first few days. Many polymorphs haven't exercised for years, and so are terribly out of shape. Move into it gradually and don't overtax your system. Most people eventually really enjoy exercising.

Week 4

DAY 1

EVALUATING YOUR PROGRESS

Every aspect of this ten-week program contributes to bringing your polymorphism under control. But none is more important than the dialogues about what you're eating and the daily phone calls to your partner. As in both of your meetings last week, you and your friend should spend part of today's session discussing your eating plans, Food Diaries, and your daily calls to your partner. Also, talk about your exercise program and the impact it has had on your well-being.

With the beginning of this fourth week, most partners really start to feel a sense of accomplishment with this program. They recognize both physiological and psychological changes and a new sense of security because they are finally stopping their overeating. Review with your partner both the small and the large changes you've noticed in your life since the beginning of this program.

In addition to discussing your successes today, talk with your partner about any difficulties you are still having. What problems have you experienced since the last meeting? Did you have one or more bingeing episodes? Have you strayed from your eating schedule without notifying your partner? What does your Food Diary reveal? Do you continue to reach for food during times of stress, fatigue, or anger? If either of you is having difficulties, agree now to support one another in a renewed effort to adhere to your program. Make a commitment to continue your eating plan, calling in, Food Diary, and exercise program every day until your next meeting.

"My biggest problem has always been late-night snacks," recalled Marjorie, a homemaker in her 40s. "For years, I would attack the refrigerator around midnight. Because my partner always went to bed at about 10:30, I used that as an excuse for not calling her when I felt the urge to have a midnight snack. I didn't want to disturb her. So instead of calling her to *talk* about these urges to binge, I would walk right past the phone to the refrigerator. There was hardly a night when I didn't stray from my eating plan."

But when Marjorie eventually talked with her friend about this problem, she made a commitment to call her partner if a crisis arose, no matter what time it was. That phone call, they agreed, absolutely *had* to be made before anything was added to or deleted from a planned menu. With the strength of this renewed pledge of support and the occasional calls, Marjorie found it easier to avoid unscheduled snacking.

"I realized that I couldn't use lateness as an excuse anymore," explains Marjorie. "I knew my partner would be there to talk if I needed her, and that seemed to boost my confidence enough to be able to handle my urges to binge. I awakened her twice to talk in those first few days, but after that I rarely had to call in the middle of the night again. I guess I just needed to know that she'd really be there whenever I needed her, and that I had her support twenty-four hours a day."

Some people have spent much of their lives overeating in a futile attempt to soothe sadness and depression, numbing the negative emotions within them. If your Food Diary has revealed that you eat during times of inner turmoil, then your partner has a particularly important role to play in the control of your overeating. After all, he, better than anyone, can empathize with some of the strong emotional needs that are driving you to food. He can give you support and understanding in any crisis you may be moving through. You should be turning to your friend, not to food, for comfort and solace.

During these opening minutes of this session, feel free to discuss any other issues with your partner, even if they don't appear to be food-related. Almost everything in your life—from problems you may be having with your boss to the rising cost of living—could be playing some role in your polymorphism. The anxieties of day-to-day life, no matter how routine or trivial they may seem at first glance, should be open topics of discussion with your partner. He or she is there to support you, not only in losing weight but in improving all aspects of your life.

DISCUSSION: SIGNIFICANT PEOPLE IN YOUR LIFE

In the first week of the program, you and your partner devoted much of your discussion time to your mother and father, talking about how you felt about them and about their feelings toward you. I would now like you and your partner to extend that discussion to the other significant people in your life—your spouse, your children, your close friends, your employer, your co-workers. Focus the conversation exclusively on how you are seen by them. What do they think of you? What is your role in their lives? What image do they have of you? All of this will, of course, be *your idea* of how they perceive you.

In this discussion, I'd like you to avoid, as much as possible, the impressions these people have of your body. For the moment, we're less concerned with how fat or thin they think you are. Other, deeper issues are usually the more significant ones that can provoke emotional turmoil within you, leading to overeating. These more meaningful themes must be confronted and understood for you to learn to respond to them in more positive ways than overeating. So concentrate on answers to such questions as:

What kind of lover/marriage partner does your lover/spouse think you are? How does he/she compliment you? How does he/she criticize you? Does your lover/spouse love you? Respect you? How do you think your lover/spouse would change you if he/she could?

If you have children, how do they evaluate you as a parent? Do they think you play too big or too small a role in their lives? Are they proud to call you "Mom" or "Dad"? What changes do you think they'd like to make in you?

How do your friends perceive you? What is your role in their lives? What traits of yours do they enjoy or find irritating? Do you ever feel you're not living up to their expectations?

Does your boss like you as an employee? As a person? What are his/her compliments and criticisms? Does he/she have confidence in your abilities and trust you to fulfill your working responsibilities?

How do your co-workers view you? Do they find you pleasant to be around? Do they compliment your skills and accomplishments or criticize you?

In this discussion, I want you to try to see the world as these other people see it. Of course, you might unintentionally be creating thoughts for them that they've never had. You may be convinced, for example, that your children think you neglect some of your parental responsibilities, but that may not be what *they* are thinking at all.

This discussion with your partner will tend to be a

reflection of *your* reality—how you perceive yourself in relation to others. So as this dialogue proceeds, constantly be evaluating whether your impressions are more yours than theirs. Do these thoughts really belong to these other people or are they really coming from you? That is, do they primarily reflect your own self-image and level of self-esteem?

In this exercise, a polymorph named Cindy told her partner, "My husband doesn't love me. When he has to stay at the office late for a business meeting, sometimes he doesn't even call to let me know. If he loved me, he wouldn't let me worry like that. He'd be thoughtful enough to call and tell me that he'll be late."

Perhaps Cindy's husband wasn't always as considerate as he might have been. But then her partner asked her, "Does he ever do anything to show he loves you?" Cindy paused a moment and then answered, "Well, I suppose he does. Over the weekend, he took me to a movie that he didn't particularly want to see, and last week he bought me flowers."

Cindy certainly wasn't keeping things in balance. She was overemphasizing the messages from her spouse that she interpreted as "he doesn't love me" and "I'm no good" while disregarding those that said "he loves me" and "he thinks I'm special." And in the process, one of her responses to this negative misconception—that she was unloved—was to binge each time her husband was late. Her self-esteem was in jeopardy, and she used food as a way of trying to soothe her hurt and frustration, and express her anger toward her husband.

Cindy's partner, however, helped her recognize a critically important fact: when her husband neglected to call, it didn't necessarily mean that he did not love her—and that she was not "worthy" of being loved—only that he was forgetful or inconsiderate that particular evening. Her husband was only human. Once Cindy clearly understood this, she no longer felt the need to eat during these times, and her bingeing episodes came to an end.

During this discussion, some polymorphs find that the thoughts they've attributed to their spouse or lover are similar to those they had ascribed to their parents three weeks earlier. "My husband belittles the value of my opinions, just like my father did," Cathy explained to her partner. "Neither of them has ever shown any confidence in my ability to do much of anything. I can sense from just the way my husband looks at me sometimes that he minimizes me as a person. And it makes me feel terrible."

This phenomenon is not surprising. After all, most of your impressions about yourself are actually coming from within you, even though they may seem to be emanating from the outside world. And psychiatrists and psychologists generally agree that these feelings toward oneself originate in childhood, usually reflecting *your ideas* of how your parents perceived you. If today you presume that your spouse, children, and friends feel a particular way about you, that is probably also how you believed your parents felt as well. Low self-esteem, then, is often based on *what you believe* are your parents' and significant others' critical or negative opinions of you.

If this discussion's relationship to your overeating is still not immediately obvious, think again about what you've read here. Perhaps you actually believe, rightly or wrongly, that your spouse, children, and others in your life really don't like you as much as you want them to, or that they think that you have some serious flaws. As I mentioned earlier, these feelings can provoke enough stress within you to send you running for comfort. Like most polymorphs, you have probably found that comfort in food.

You will learn here to change your behavior and begin positively confronting and dealing with these ideas. Most likely, until now you've simply integrated them into your belief system, where they've settled into your unconscious mind. You may binge on a bag of cookies after a confrontation with your husband or mother and never really understand the connection between your self-image and your overeating. But how you see yourself can dramatically influence your behavior. To soothe the pain of your anxieties and insecurities, you overeat—usually without even realizing why. You tranquilize your pain with food. And it becomes a vicious cycle. The anxiety causes you to eat and gain weight, which creates even more anxiety, and, in turn, more overeating and weight gain.

In your discussions with your partner, be sensitive to issues involving low self-esteem. Become an "active listener"; let your partner bounce his ideas and thoughts off you and help him keep them in proper perspective. Restate what he is saying and help him organize his thoughts so he can see them more clearly. For example: "Cindy, you're telling me how your husband neglected or forgot to call you last night. You haven't really told me, though, how he doesn't love you. If I were in your place, I might be thinking about whether I just felt unlovable or unworthy of his love."

Once these issues are out in the open, you and your partner can begin discussing and evaluating them. It is important for you to recognize that your misperceptions of the behavior of others may be causing you to overeat. With your partner you can start dealing more honestly and clearly with these issues in order to finally resolve them.

Continue this discussion about your spouse, children, friends, and boss for the remainder of the meeting. Use the insights you acquire to help modify your sense of the world. No one is perfect, nor do they need to be perfect to prove their love and respect for each other. Overeating to compensate for your own or another person's imperfections is obviously ineffective and may well be one of the reasons for your polymorphism.

This discussion will form the foundation for a psychodrama, or role-playing exercise, that you and your partner will participate in at the next meeting. The psychodrama, too, will help you understand your relationships with other people and how they influence your behavior.

EXERCISING

Spend fifteen minutes of today's meeting exercising with your partner. One week has passed since you and your partner began exercising daily and, like other polymorphs, your reaction to it may range from excitement to resistance. Some polymorphs, accustomed to a sedentary life, find it difficult to get their bodies moving. If that's the case with you, renew your commitment to stick with exercising. You will find that not only will it soon become easier, but it will also be more fulfilling as the days pass.

After a couple of weeks of exercise, some polymorphs find physical activity so exhilarating that they actually want to *expand* their fitness regimen. As a first step, try adding some walking to your daily schedule. A woman named Suzanne recently stopped relying on her car to run errands. The supermarket was only three blocks from her house, so she began walking there and back. She would also wake up half an hour before her family in the morning and spend thirty minutes walking through the neighborhood. She and her partner agreed to engage in at least one activity together each week that would require some walking—including strolls through parks, museums, and art galleries.

Even when exercise seems like a difficult, time-consuming intrusion into your day, keep in mind that it is an efficient stress-reducer and can help relieve the frustration that can make you want to overeat.

DAY 2

EVALUATING YOUR PROGRESS

Often, at this stage of the program, polymorphs tell me that they're beginning to have some problems contending with the advice of family members in relation to this program, and that they may even feel the urge to overeat in these situations. One woman, for instance, recalls her difficulty coping with her husband's continuous suggestions of "better ways" to lose weight "even faster," such as:

> "Why don't you try that new protein diet that my secretary is on?"
>
> "If you're really serious about losing weight, why don't you just eliminate sweets from now on?"

Comments like these typically come from mates who may feel anxious about some aspect of this program. Although they love you, they may unconsciously be trying to sabotage this program. Perhaps they're becoming jealous of the close relationship you are forming with your partner, fearful that it may cause some marital conflict. Or maybe they're anxious that you may be revealing "family secrets" to your friend. Or perhaps they're uneasy with the early loss of weight that you might already have achieved. For some people, any change in the family system—even positive change like weight loss—is unsettling. They are familiar and comfortable with their lives as they are and unconsciously would prefer to leave things unaltered—even unpleasant things—rather than having to learn to adapt to change. The fear of the unknown is often much more threatening than an unsatisfactory status quo.

If friends or family members are becoming a detriment

to your program, discuss this with your partner now. Remember that your decision-making process in relation to this program no longer involves only you—it is now an interaction between you and your partner, so in deciding how to deal with this situation, your friend should play a role.

Based on experience with many patients, I usually suggest that polymorphs not take up this issue directly with their family members yet. You will do that later in the program. For now, try to understand what is happening by discussing with your partner the possible unconscious sabotage by your family. And as one means of resisting this sabotage, commit yourself to the program one day at a time. Instead of worrying about what might happen with your spouse, child, or parent tomorrow or next week, or feeling bad about problems that may have occurred yesterday, stay in the present. Devote your energy to making *today's* eating plan work; don't focus on the past or future behavior of a family member. Many people become so preoccupied with anxieties related to the past or future that they never recognize that today—at this very moment—their life is actually very good. Allow yourself to enjoy and make the most of the present.

Also take a few minutes here to discuss with your partner other relevant issues, including your progress with the eating plan and the calling-in system, the Food Diary, and the exercise program. The Food Diary will probably be showing a pattern of stabilized behavior by now. Discuss the diary and congratulate yourselves on your progress.

PSYCHODRAMA

At the last meeting, you and your partner talked about how you think you are perceived by the significant people in your life. Discussions like that are important, because people tend to imagine that everyone else perceives life as they do. Consequently, we expect our friends and family to fully understand and be sensitive to our periods of hurt, pain, love, passion, anger, and anxiety. But no one, not even a twin brother or sister, sees the world exactly as we do. Everyone has different experiences, and thus has a unique point of view from which he perceives his environment.

Today's exercise is designed to help you understand this concept better and gain greater insight into how the people closest to you see you and your polymorphism. Both now and during your next meeting, you and your partner will try to put yourselves inside the heads of the most important people in your lives. For a few minutes you will, in effect, *become* these persons, seeing the world through their eyes. In a psychodrama, a husband can become a wife, a parent can become a child, a woman can become a man, and vice versa, simply by attempting to think, speak, and behave like that person.

Before beginning, you and your partner should decide which one of you will become the main subject of today's psychodrama. The other will have center stage during the next meeting. The two of you will be participating in the psychodrama both days, but only one person will be the primary focus of attention each time. If you have more than one partner, each psychodrama should be conducted in front of the entire group; an extra meeting or two should be scheduled so each member can have a turn.

Let's assume that you and your partner have decided that you—the reader of this book—will be the principal subject today. To get started, you should list the significant people in your own life. These are the people who make up your environment and could be playing a role in your polymorphism—spouse or lover, parent(s), child(ren), friends, employer, coworkers. During the rest of this session, you will deal with some or all of these people, one by one.

Then take two chairs, place them facing each other, and seat yourselves in them. Next, I'd like your partner to ask you questions designed to provoke insights into your relationship with the first of the significant people that you've listed—say, your spouse. Because the two of you have already had several hours of discussion, your partner probably knows enough about your husband or wife to formulate his own questions. But if he needs some help, here are some areas you can profitably explore:

How does your spouse (lover, child, parent, etc.) generally feel toward you?

What does he/she like about you?

What does he/she dislike about you?

Does this person truly love and/or respect you?

Does this person make you feel worthwhile?

What was the last conflict in which the two of you engaged?

Was this conflict handled and resolved fairly?

What are his/her feelings toward your polymorphism?

Did this person treat you differently when you weighed less?

After you've briefly answered all of your partner's questions, the two of you should change seats and then, as realistically as possible, I'd like you (Polymorph #1) to "become" your spouse, or the person you were just discussing, and your partner (Polymorph #2) to "become" *you*. He will begin directing questions at you once again, but this time each of you will be playing your new roles. You will respond to his questions as your spouse. So your partner (playing you) might ask:

What's your general attitude toward me?

What do you like about me?

What do you dislike about me?

Do you think our last conflict was handled and resolved fairly?

What are your feelings toward my weight?

Once again, in answering these questions, your responsibility is to answer them as though you were your spouse. Respond instinctively and rapidly, without giving yourself a chance to intellectualize. Your partner should interrupt and correct you if you start replying, "Well, I think my spouse, Joe, would say . . ." She should guide you by saying, "I'm not interested in what Linda thinks; I'm talking to *you* now, Joe. Joe, tell me how *you* feel." Answer spontaneously and directly as your spouse would: "I really don't like all the fat you've gained in the last ten years." Concentrate on *becoming* your spouse. See yourself as really being him, speaking the very words that he would. As you respond, your partner should answer just as *you* might (for example, "I'm making an honest effort to lose weight now"), and a dialogue can begin, letting the conversation flow in whatever direction it naturally moves. It will happen much more easily than you might think.

Your polymorphism need not be the subject of this psychodrama, as there may be other relevant issues that you'd like to deal with here. (The most recent argument you had with your spouse or other family member is usually a good psychodrama subject.) But in many cases, your weight will be a central issue of conflict, particularly between spouses and other family members.

When Linda and her partner, Suzanne, switched roles—with Linda portraying her husband and Suzanne playing Linda—the women made an honest attempt to delve into the feelings behind the issue of polymorphism:

SUZANNE (AS LINDA): "Even when you don't pick on my

weight, I really feel it's always in the back of your mind. I don't think that's fair."

LINDA (AS HER HUSBAND): "I haven't thought about or mentioned your weight in weeks."

SUZANNE (AS LINDA): "What about two nights ago, when you came home early and said, 'Oh . . . isn't dinner ready yet?' I'm very sensitive to that. I get the feeling that you think I'm just a fat person who does nothing else all day but spend time in the kitchen cooking and eating."

LINDA (AS HER HUSBAND): "Honey, you're oversensitive. I simply asked you about dinner. Please don't read anything into what I'm saying. You know me—if I really had something more on my mind, I would have come right out and said it."

Linda, in trying to see her family situation from her husband's point of view, recognized through this exercise that she did sometimes overreact to things her husband said. Being so sensitive about her obesity, she probably often misinterpreted others' innocent remarks.

Before beginning this exercise, a polymorph named Rod told his partner, Jeffrey, "I really don't think my wife loves me as much as she used to. We fight all the time, usually about how much I eat. She must be embarrassed by the way I look, and I feel that I've let her down by not getting my weight under control. I don't blame her for not loving me."

When Rod and Jeffrey switched roles, they decided to delve into this issue of love, and midway through the psychodrama, the conversation proceeded this way:

ROD (AS HIS WIFE): "You're right, I don't like you overweight. But that's a totally separate issue from love. I get angry at you and I worry about you, but I've never stopped loving you because you weigh more."

JEFFREY (AS ROD): "Then why is it such a big issue with you? If you love me, why can't you just accept me as I am?"

ROD (AS HIS WIFE): "I always love you. But I *like* you better thin. Maybe it's my hangup, but when you're skinny, you're much more appealing to me. But I don't love you any less now than I ever did."

JEFFREY (AS ROD): "So you really love me? I've had my doubts. Do you really love me?"

ROD (AS HIS WIFE): "Yes, I love you."

This dialogue may seem simplistic as you read it. But most partners are surprised at how easily they can assume the attitudes and true feelings of the people in their lives, and make statements that contradict what they had thought the attitudes of others would actually be.

However, sometimes the psychodramas aren't resolved as pleasantly as Rod's. When Barbara assumed the role of her husband, she found him saying, "You know, I do find your obesity obnoxious. I really do. I can't stand it. I've told you this a thousand times. Your fatness is ugly."

Barbara cried during this exercise, but as difficult as it was for her, she felt better after having gone through it. Now that she was clearer than ever about where her husband stood, her own determination to control her compulsive disease increased.

"My husband's feelings are disturbing to me, and they really hurt me each time I hear them," Barbara explained later. "But when I spoke those words as if they were coming out of his mouth, I really had to face it like never before. I now know that this is something I have to overcome, and I see that very plainly. I'm not as afraid to deal with it as I once was."

Near the end of this first psychodrama, switch roles once more, with you portraying yourself again and your partner playing your spouse. At this time, you may want to engage your "spouse" in a dialogue based upon the new insights you've gained. In a sense, this may be a "behavioral rehearsal" for what you'll actually be telling your real spouse later in the day. Because you'll have already rehearsed it here and have prepared what you're going to say and what the responses are likely to be, your own anxiety will be minimal at that time. You'll feel in control and the entire process will become easier for you.

For example, after the psychodrama that placed her so closely in touch with her husband's negative feelings about her obesity, Barbara switched roles and, as herself, told her partner (playing her husband): "I understand that you don't feel good about my fatness. But I have a disease, and I'm doing something to control it. It would be nice if you'd read this book so you'd know what my problem is and what I'm doing about it. I'm not popping diet pills or going on some wacky diet; I'm really working hard to try to control this problem. I'm sorry I'm a polymorph, but I am."

Later that night, Barbara told her husband exactly that. And because Barbara presented the issue so clearly and matter-of-factly, her husband responded positively, and even offered to support his wife in whatever way he could.

Ralph, immediately following a psychodrama that examined his relationship with his son, felt in a very loving, compromising mood. He had asked his partner to portray his son, and then apologized to the boy for the conflicts in their lives in recent years. This family dissension had caused almost constant stress in Ralph's life, to which he reacted by overeating, drowning his anxiety in food. The day after the psychodrama, however, Ralph told his son about the exercise and apologized for their difficulties. He and his son had the warmest, most sincere conversation they had had in years, and that was the forerunner to other similar conversations in the future. As Ralph grew closer to his son, the anxiety in his life was reduced and he eventually stopped "needing" food to comfort him.

For as long as time allows, move through as many of the other people on your list as possible in this meeting. Be flexible; if you find you're spending thirty or forty minutes on a particular person, that's fine. It is not essential that everyone on your list be dealt with at this meeting. In fact, you and your partner might wish to schedule an additional meeting this week to take care of the issues and people left untouched here, or you might repeat the exercise at an upcoming meeting when you can extend the length of the session. Don't rush through the psychodrama process; it can be very revealing and useful if you allow yourself to become immersed in it.

The psychodrama exercise can help you to see that there may be a difference between reality and how you perceive it. By looking at the world through the eyes of your spouse, lover, parents, or children, you may gain some insight into your relationship with these individuals. You'll examine issues—including your overweight problem—from completely different points of view than you may be accustomed to. You will look closely at how others feel about you and how you can best respond to these feelings. And in the process, you will practice confronting emotional problems more constructively, instead of using food as comfort.

Incidentally, I've provided you with many of the tools you need to effectively perform the psychodrama. But if you want to learn more about this technique, I suggest you read Dr. Lewis Yablonsky's book, *Psychodrama*.

EXERCISING

Spend fifteen minutes of today's meeting moving through your exercises with your partner. You may have been surprised to notice by now that physical activity actually *decreases* your hunger rather than increases it. In study after study, physiologists have shown that when you keep your body in shape through moderate exercise you maximize the efficiency of all of your physiological processes, including the proper regulation of your hunger mechanism. By contrast, when you lead a sedentary life, the body's functioning is thrown off-balance, and you will tend to eat more than you really need to meet your body's energy requirements. Exercising regularly, then, gives you an extra tool in your arsenal against compulsive overeating.

Although there is probably no need for you to continue keeping the Food Diary (you should have a good understanding of your eating behavior by now), for next week's meeting, it's necessary to continue the other major aspects of the program, including the eating plan, the daily calling in, and a daily exercise routine.

Week 5

DAY 1

EVALUATING YOUR PROGRESS

In this session with your partner, spend ten to fifteen minutes discussing your progress and problems with the food program, the calling-in system, and the daily exercising. These critically important ingredients in controlling your polymorphism must be talked about and monitored at every meeting. Some partners arrive at these sessions with a list of subjects they would like to discuss.

During this dialogue, some polymorphs share their excitement about the growing ease with which they are able to abide by their daily food plan. While in the beginning it may have been difficult for them to follow their prearranged menu without frequent lapses, their bingeing is usually now under more control, and they feel capable of taking charge of their compulsive overeating.

This is also your opportunity, of course, to talk about any difficulties you are experiencing. For instance, have you had problems contacting your partner by phone for your daily sharing of menus? Are you feeling any resistance about coming to meetings? Do you find yourself still eating compulsively when you're bored or feeling insecure? How is your family encouraging or limiting your progress?

During this part of the meeting, Charles discussed the uncontrollable eating binges that occurred whenever he was fatigued, particularly after returning home from work. He had a pressure-packed job as an advertising executive, and when his workday ended he would cope with his physical and mental weariness by going to the refrigerator and snacking until dinner. Then he would eat a large, full meal.

After talking with his partner about this chronic problem, Charles agreed to phone his friend immediately upon arriving home each evening. This call was to be his first action when he walked in the door. During these early-evening phone calls, he and his partner would talk about Charles' fatigue and how he could relieve it *without* overeating—by taking a soothing shower, enjoying a nap, or relaxing on his patio with a book. Often, merely by talking with his partner, Charles felt such a sense of warmth, comfort, and support that the urge to binge disappeared for the rest of the evening.

Be as honest as you can with your partner in these discussions. As you have probably recognized by now, most of the embarrassment you had anticipated feeling in this program never materialized. There is nothing to be ashamed of if you still occasionally binge or if you continue to have problems in separating eating from activities like watching TV. If you stick to this program, you *will* eventually gain control of these problem areas, whether you accomplish it in the first or the tenth week.

SECOND PSYCHODRAMA

For most of the remainder of today's meeting, you and your partner will continue the psychodrama that you began in the last session. This time, the focus should move to the other person—that is, if you were the center of attention at the previous meeting, your partner should step into the spotlight today.

Follow the same procedure as last time. Have your partner (if he is the principal subject of this psychodrama) verbally list the significant people in his life—spouse, parent(s), child(ren), friends, employer, co-workers. Then he should deal with as many of them as possible, one by one, trying to gain insights into any conflicts with them and probing how they could be influencing his polymorphism.

As in the last meeting, the two of you should be seated opposite one another. Your partner should select one of the people on his list, and then you should begin asking him questions about this particular individual: What is the general attitude of this person toward you? What recent conflicts have you had? Have they been handled and resolved fairly? And so on.

Then change seats and, as you do, switch roles—that is, you will now portray your partner while he plays the significant person he has just been discussing. Once again, ask him a series of questions; this time he should answer them from the point of view of this other person.

Few polymorphs fail to find some value in this experience. Each of us relates to the people in our environment in a particular manner, and by reversing roles you will possibly understand other individuals' thoughts, feelings, and behaviors better than ever before as you try to identify with them and see the world as they do. Your attitudes toward these people can change in just a few minutes, and you may begin to discover a means of resolving conflicts that have persisted for months or even years. As these problems disappear, the anxiety that accompanied them will vanish as well. If this stress contributed to your overeating by driving you to food for comfort, the psychodrama can become an important process in controlling your polymorphism.

You may also discover that during the psychodrama, you may transcend the denial system you have hidden behind for so long. For years, you may have distorted not only your own reality, but also the way you imagined others were reacting to you. But during role-reversal, because it is something new, you will tend to let your defenses drop as you experiment with it and test out its potential and its limits. While playing another person, you'll be approaching the subject matter from an entirely new point of view—one that is not encumbered by rationalizations and defenses that have developed over many years. Your responses—if you allow them to be spontaneous and intuitive—will be honest and direct.

For example, I recall a recent psychodrama in which a polymorph named Karla was extremely concerned about regaining the weight she had already lost. "My boyfriend is so happy about my shedding so many pounds; I just know that if I regain the weight, I might lose him," she explained. Karla was aware of how anxious this worrying made her, and how this self-aggravation might someday even cause her to binge.

In a psychodrama, when she and her partner, Jane, assumed new roles, she realized that her fears were probably unfounded. Thirty minutes into their psychodrama, as Karla became comfortable playing the role of Don, the following exchange occurred:

JANE (AS KARLA): "I've lost a lot of weight, Don, and I know how happy that makes you. You compliment me a lot, and even tell your friends how successful I've been in this program. Well, I'm scared now about disappointing you. Every time I've ever lost weight in my life, I've always gained it back, and more. I'm just afraid it's going to happen again, and I don't want it to. I think it might make you unhappy and embarrassed if I start putting on weight again. And in the back of my mind, I'm thinking that you might even leave me if that happens."

KARLA (AS DON): "Well, I like you better thin, Karla. I think you're sexier and more attractive that way."

JANE (AS KARLA): "But what would happen if I regained the weight? Would you be angry?"

KARLA (AS DON): "Maybe a part of me would. But, Karla, I know how hard you're trying with this program. I'm supporting you, and Jane's supporting you, and I don't think you're going to slip that much. I've told you that I'm behind you 100 percent, haven't I?"

JANE (AS KARLA): "Yes. But I just need to know that you'll be behind me through the bad times as well as the good."

KARLA (AS DON): "I've given you my word on that already. You've trusted me on everything else in our relationship. Trust me on this, too."

Through the psychodrama, Karla brought Don's, as well as her own, feelings into clearer awareness, clarifying her understanding of their relationship, particularly in relation to her polymorphism.

Although psychodrama may help you better perceive the thoughts and feelings of others, it might also make you aware of just how inattentive you've been to those around you, because of your preoccupation with your weight. During a role-reversal, Bill assumed the role of his son, and when his partner asked him some pointed questions about their father-son relationship, Bill often responded, "I really don't know how I [my son] feel about that. My dad and I have never talked about it."

In the psychodrama, Bill recognized how poorly he had communicated with his son. "We hardly ever talked," Bill recalled later, "and when we did, I usually did the talking, most often yelling at him for something he had done wrong." That day, Bill practiced with his partner communicating with his son, and made a commitment to become closer to his boy. In the weeks that followed, as his relationship with his son improved, Bill's overeating compulsions diminished, indicating that some of his eating may have been a response to family anxieties.

As you and your partner move through this second experience with psychodrama, refer back a few pages for more detailed guidelines on how the session should proceed. But don't allow yourself to become too constrained; follow any subject matter that either of you feels is important, even if it seems unrelated to polymorphism.

During her psychodrama, Lisa chose to spend some time acting out a job interview with a prospective employer. She was determined to find a new job, but was nervous about the interviewing process. So, with her partner playing a potential employer and Lisa playing herself, they spent thirty minutes "rehearsing" the interview. This experience boosted Lisa's self-confidence by allowing her to practice responding to the questions she would probably be asked.

Lisa got the job. She said later that the interview was "easy," and that at times, she felt that the interviewer was more nervous than her, since she had already "experienced" the interview with her partner.

EXERCISING

During today's session, spend a few minutes exercising with your partner. As you are finding out, physical exercise does not have to be terribly strenuous to enhance your physical well-being and your self-esteem. Today, try to add an extra three to five repetitions to each exercise you perform.

You can also incorporate new forms of physical activity into your regular schedule. The more you exercise, the better you will feel and the more weight you will lose.

DAY 2

EVALUATING YOUR PROGRESS

As usual, begin today's meeting with a discussion of your progress with this program. You and your partner are now at the halfway point in this ten-week plan, and you should take a hard look at exactly where you are. In a few minutes, the two of you will weigh and measure yourselves, which will provide you with concrete evidence of how your body is doing. But be careful not to place too much emphasis on these results. More importantly, concentrate on the program itself. Is everything running smoothly? Are there any problems with your food plan, the calling-in system, or your exercising? Talk about any setbacks either of you may have experienced, and support each other in overcoming these obstacles.

At this stage in the program, polymorphs sometimes find themselves with feelings of deprivation during the day:

"The hardest thing for me is not having a doughnut during the coffee break at work. Everyone around me is eating one, and I feel deprived."

"Now that I've cut out dessert from my dinner, I really miss it. I never realized how important it was to me."

Offer each other encouragement and strength to move through any feelings of deprivation. Everyone experiences problems now and then, but you have your partner to emotionally nourish you during your difficult times.

WEIGHING AND MEASURING

Almost a month has passed since you and your partner started this program, and it's time to weigh and measure yourselves for the second time. Do it now, recording the results on the chart you used during the first meeting.

By this point in the program, most polymorphs are eager to discover how much weight they've actually lost. The chances are that gradual weight loss has been occurring, and that there are also positive changes in your measurements—hips, waist, etc. Don't forget, however, that everyone is different. Some people lose pounds and inches faster than others.

So don't become discouraged if your partner is having more dramatic and more visible results than you.

This weighing-and-measuring session is only a progress report. The next time you take out the scale and tape measure—which will be in the tenth week—the physical results should be even more encouraging. But more than simply losing weight and knowing that they look better, many polymorphs tell me that the weigh-in also offers them concrete proof of having gained control over their lives.

"I have been feeling better about myself since this program started," explained Elaine. "I've come to see myself more objectively—as a person with a weight problem who also happens to have some very nice qualities."

BODY AWARENESS AND RELAXATION

Many overweight people feel alienated from their bodies: they avoid looking at themselves. Now that you are losing weight, however, your attitude has probably begun to gradually change.

Spend a few minutes talking with your partner about how your feelings toward your physical self have been altered in the last five weeks. Were you estranged from your body before you began this program? Did you feel self-conscious when other people glanced at you? How differently do you feel today? Has your loss of weight affected your body image? Has your daily exercising helped you become attuned to your body in a positive manner?

After you and your partner have discussed your body and your evolving relationship with it, I'd like to introduce you to a simple relaxation technique that you should start practicing every day. Like daily exercising, relaxation can promote positive feelings about yourself and your body, and help relieve the stress that often causes polymorphs to overeat. It will teach you just how easily you can assert control over your body in just a few minutes.

There are dozens of relaxation techniques, and most have produced amazing results. I'd like to introduce you now to a relaxation method that I've found particularly effective for polymorphs, adapted from a program developed by Dr. C. Norman Shealy in his book, *90 Days to Self-Health.* For the next few minutes, I would like both you and your partner to practice this technique. Have your partner read it aloud, slowly, as you lie in a prone position and proceed through it. Then you should do the same for him.

Begin by allowing your body to be completely relaxed. Lean back . . . rest your arms beside you . . . and close your eyes. . . . Keep your eyes closed gently, while you learn to relax.

I take a deep breath and hold it . . . now I let it out slowly. . . . I take another deep breath and hold it. . . . I let it out slowly; I feel the tightness going out of my chest and body.

I now focus my attention on my hands; I notice the feelings from them and let go of the muscles; I relax the muscles in my hands.

I let the relaxation begin to flow from the muscles of my fingers and hands . . . up through my wrists . . . and into my forearms. I feel my forearms getting looser and heavier.

I let go now in my upper arms. . . . The relaxation is moving from muscle to muscle. . . . A pleasantly heavy feeling is coming into my arms.

Now I let the relaxation move up through my shoulders and into my neck. . . . I let the muscles in my neck slacken.

I pay attention to my scalp. . . . I let the muscles become loose and limp. . . . I smooth out my forehead; I imagine it getting smooth and relaxed. . . . The heavy feeling is flowing down across my face. . . . I relax the muscles around my eyes. . . . I relax my cheeks. . . . My jaw muscles and the muscles around my mouth are also getting heavier and more relaxed.

The relaxation is now flowing down into my chest. . . . I enjoy the sensation. . . . I notice now the muscles in my abdomen. . . . I feel these muscles getting looser. . . . Now I relax the muscles in my back, my upper and lower back. . . . All the tightness is leaving my back.

The muscles around my hips and thighs are getting looser and more relaxed. . . . I can feel the wave of relaxation spreading down through my chest, stomach, and hips. The relaxation is deep . . . deeper and deeper. . . . I let the relaxation flow down my legs . . . through my knees . . . now into my calves. . . . I relax the muscles in my feet. . . . I let my feet get relaxed.

My whole body is still getting more relaxed. . . . I tune in to any part of my body where there may still be some tightness. . . . I just think of relaxing those parts, and I find that they become much more relaxed than they now are. . . . I continue relaxing. I enjoy it.

At the end of the exercise, open your eyes slowly and give yourself a few seconds to reorient yourself to the surroundings. You may be surprised at how serene you feel. Let yourself enjoy the experience, and get in touch with just how much pleasure your body—which has been your antagonist for so many years—can give you.

I suggest that you make your own tape recording of the above exercise and listen to it as you practice the exercise, at least once a day, for five to ten minutes. By making it part of your life, you can help keep your stress under control and, in turn, minimize the number of anxiety-related eating episodes.

EXERCISING

During today's session, you and your partner should exercise together. You both should persistently adhere to this part of the ten-week plan. Exercise is a simple and relatively painless way to tone up your body as it adjusts to your decreasing weight. It is also a means of stimulating additional weight loss without further changes in your eating plan.

I recall a patient named Pat, who said, "I had been on dozens of diets in the past, and one of the things they all had in common was that losing weight became more difficult with each pound lost. The interesting thing about exercise, though, is that it becomes *easier* with each passing day. The first few times I exercised it was tough, but it gradually became less of a strain, and soon I was enjoying it. It was another activity that my partner and I could do together, and this sharing brought us even closer together."

Once again, I suggest that in addition to your daily exercise regimen, please take advantage of the dozens of other opportunities during the week to physically challenge yourself a little. Walk, rather than drive, as much as possible. Climb a flight of stairs instead of riding an elevator. And even if you don't add any new activities to your physical-fitness regimen now, recommit yourself to regularly sharing with your partner the exercises that you have planned in this program.

Week 6

DAY 1

EVALUATING YOUR PROGRESS

Spend a few minutes here discussing with your partner the successes and slips you've each had since the last meeting in regard to your respective food plans, the calling-in system, and daily exercising. I'm sure you are constantly seeing signs of improvement as your excess pounds steadily disappear. You may notice, for example, that you have some extra energy during certain times of the day when you never had it before. While there still may be occasional regressions with this program, by now you are learning how to react to them constructively by calling your partner for help. Talking about your food-related problems is the key to handling both the urge to eat and the causes behind that craving.

BLOCKS TO SUCCESS: BINGEING

There are many common blocks to weight-loss success, from internal resistances to external subversions. In the external environment, there are dozens of social cues for eating, from food advertising, to social gatherings where binge foods proliferate, to scores of fast-food restaurants constantly beckoning you. By now, I hope you understand the power of these environmental cues and have learned how to neutralize them. If you're still having problems, I suggest you reacquaint yourself with some of the techniques described in Week 2. For example, some polymorphs tell me they avoid overeating at social events by making a conscientious effort to chew very slowly and deliberately, allowing their appestat to be activated before they have eaten more food than they really want to. Also, most overeaters discover that they can successfully deal with the temptation of food advertising by firmly adhering to their prearranged menus and the calling-in program, using their partner for support during any weak moments.

The internal, subconscious resistances to success with this program are more abstract than the external temptations, and are often more difficult to cope with. Much of this entire program, however, is designed to help you comprehend and overcome them. One woman, for instance, told me that she believed her binges resulted from her own insecurity about dealing with all the new challenges that her thinness would present—from new social relationships to more desirable job opportunities. Her poor self-esteem, then, was her biggest obstacle to permanently losing weight. Throughout this ten-week plan, however, you and your partner are learning about your own worthiness, and, gradually, your increased self-assurance will allow you to more confidently face and successfully manage almost any situation. When that happens, your bingeing episodes will decrease significantly.

But no matter how successful this program is, compulsive overeaters can still expect food binges to surface occasionally in response to emotions (frustration, anger, depression, sadness) that the polymorph has for years tried to soothe by eating. If you habitually overeat whenever you're angry at your boss, jealous of a lover, or worried about a teenage daughter staying out too late on Saturday night, that kind of chronic behavior won't change overnight.

"My biggest concern was that I wanted to loose all my extra pounds immediately," recalls Margaret, who had a history of bingeing whenever she was particularly anxious. "Even though I seemed to be losing steadily—my clothes were gradually getting looser—that wasn't fast enough for me at first. Eventually, this frustration made me so tense that to cope, I would eat."

Margaret discussed this behavior with her partner and realized that this behavior was sabotaging her program. Whenever she felt the anxiety of wanting to lose weight faster, she would immediately pick up the phone. With her friend's support—and particularly since her partner revealed that she, too, had the same frustration—Margaret and her partner eventually learned to accept *gradual* weight loss. With her anxiety eased, Margaret found herself less tempted to binge.

A woman named Beverly changed the way that she had reacted to binges for years. "In the past, whenever I would overeat in the middle of a diet," she recalls, "I would use that as an excuse for dropping out of the program completely. I used to tell myself, 'This isn't going to work for me; I'm just going to give up and accept the fact that I'll always be overweight.'

"But now, instead of talking to myself that way, I talk to my partner, and the outcome is a lot better. My friend and I always come to the conclusion that my occasional binges are problems that everyone has, and that I am quite capable of managing them before they get totally out of control."

In addition, like many other compulsive overeaters, Beverly discovered that she could control her food consumption more easily when food wasn't so readily accessible. Many men and women in this ten-week program tell me that when they shop in the supermarket they feel obligated to buy certain food items, like ice cream or cookies, for the sake of the rest of the family. In fact, however, your family members would probably also benefit from a reduction or elimination of sweets and other fattening foods in their own diets, even if they are not overweight. If they must occasionally satisfy their sweet tooth, they can buy and consume their sugar outside the home, where it won't tempt you.

One polymorph told her family members, "I'm not being fair to myself by having binge food around. We'd probably all be better off if none of us ever had them, but if you feel *you* need them, please buy and eat them outside the house. That's how you can support me."

On the other hand, when polymorphs find that their program is going well, they may become overly confident and start ignoring various aspects of it. The calling-in system is often the first component to be neglected. Talk with your partner about any tendency in either of you to slight it. Urge one another to move past the resistances when they occur, and make the phone calls. Each time the two of you report your respective menus to one another, you are helping to continue your commitment to specific food choices and a sensible style of eating. The calling-in plan must be an essential part of your daily routine. Continuing it will help make your newly acquired habits part of your life.

So while no one is immune to bingeing, this program offers you the best possible chance for realizing control over the self-destructive eating episodes because it is a comprehensive assault on both the psychological and physical aspects of your overeating. Despite occasional slips, you can achieve long-term results as you explore, understand, and deal with the various external and internal cues that can trigger a binge.

A COMMITMENT TO PLAY

The three essential elements of life are generally acknowledged to be love, work, and play. As adults, however, few of us spend enough time on purely pleasurable activities. Too many people believe that play is essentially a childhood diversion that has little place in life beyond adolescence.

Not so. Everyone deserves—and requires—pleasure and play in their life. Many researchers have documented the staggering rate of change in our society and the resulting overload of stress, from tension over the economy to job problems. Polymorphs, however, are affected not only by the everyday stresses of modern living but also by the anxieties associated with being overweight—by the anger, frustration, and depression they feel in relation to their eating habits and their bodies. Even though it is almost impossible to instantly remove these stressors from your life, you *can* periodically remove *yourself* from your stressful environment for a few hours at a time, through pleasurable, relaxing activity.

Today, I want you and your partner to make a commitment to do something enjoyable and purely selfish for yourselves for two hours a week.

Whatever you choose, make it a specific activity and allow yourself to be thoroughly absorbed in it for those two hours a week, to relish the experience completely, banishing thoughts of whatever else you "should be doing instead." By the time you get back to your responsibilities, you'll feel refreshed, relaxed, and better able to cope with everyday tensions.

Spend twenty to thirty minutes now talking with your partner about what you enjoy doing, but never seem to allow yourself the time to do. Plan to escape for two hours a week, or for even more time if you wish. Try to choose activities you can do together—perhaps swimming at a health spa or reading in the sun. Permit yourselves to be nourished with fun.

EXERCISE/RELAXATION

In your last meeting, you and your partner were introduced to a relaxation technique. This type of silent, passive relaxation method is an excellent way of coping with the life stresses discussed above. It will slow down the bodily processes, quiet the mind, and help you rid yourself of anxieties. Used in conjunction with your daily exercising, the relaxation technique will promote positive feelings about your body as well as facilitate good health. Thus I believe that both are important to continue on a regular basis. One should not replace the other.

So within each of your biweekly sessions with your partner, the two of you should integrate both of these activities. As a general rule, most polymorphs find that the physical exercises work best at the very beginning of the meeting and the relaxation technique at the end. This is the regimen I suggest, but wherever you decide to schedule them during the meeting, make certain that both are part of every session. Also, don't neglect these two components during your nonmeeting days. You should do both the exercises and the relaxation technique on your own during the days when you and your partner aren't getting together.

DAY 2

EVALUATING YOUR PROGRESS

In the opening minutes of today's meeting, talk with your partner about what you have been eating, the calling-in system, exercising, and the relaxation technique. Share your positive experiences, including your growing ability to adhere to your prearranged menu. Occasional setbacks are perfectly normal and expected, but by now the momentum of your weeks of success with the program should be carrying you past those difficult times.

"A few years ago, when I was moving from one gimmicky diet to the next, I was obsessed with food," recalled Mary. "I would eat breakfast and then count the minutes until I could eat carrot sticks for lunch. The same clock-watching would continue until dinner. I'd also spend a lot of time sifting through a shoebox of recipes and diets to decide which one I'd try next. But this ten-week program settled me down. I became secure with it, and food stopped becoming such a preoccupation in my life. When that happened, I started losing weight, and I've never regained it."

Share your own experiences—both successes and failures—with your partner now.

BLOCKS TO SUCCESS: FAMILY AND SIDE ISSUES

For the next thirty to forty minutes, discuss with your partner the major obstacles that still stand between you and complete success with this program. At the last meeting, I suggested that the two of you talk about bingeing, which for many polymorphs is the most serious problem they must overcome at this point of the ten-week plan. Now spend some time exploring other areas where difficulties commonly persist, such as family-related problems and various side issues that can divert you from dealing intently with your compulsive overeating.

Family (or Roommate) Problems

When polymorphs begin this program, most have the support of the people close to them, including spouses, children, lovers, roommates, and parents. But that enthusiasm sometimes wanes, and ironically this usually occurs about midway through the ten weeks, when the program is clearly beginning to work. The motivation behind many supporters-turned-saboteurs is actually understandable. For instance, family members may grumble about your revised eating and cooking habits—these quite naturally become a bore for people who don't need to lose weight. Consider also the impatience and even irritation that could result from hearing you constantly talk about your sessions with your partner. As loving and concerned as those close to you may be, only another polymorph can fully understand what you're going through.

Almost all family sabotage occurs unconsciously on the part of the saboteur. For example, I've mentioned several times how roommates or family members may subvert the polymorph's success because of their own anxieties about changes in their relationships. A patient named Steve discovered that his roommate (also a polymorph) became resentful because their shared activity of eating had ended. So, quite unconsciously, he began sabotaging Steve's program, offering occasional midnight snacks and suggesting that "a day off from your eating plan isn't going to hurt."

I have described the weight-loss saboteur frequently in this book, and will discuss this phenomenon again in Week 9. But for now, because there may be subtle ways that your program is being undermined, it's important that you understand the role that the saboteur may be unconsciously playing as a block to your success. Although only rarely will people deliberately try to keep you overweight, their negative behavior can nevertheless create stress and cause you to overeat.

Whenever you encounter family sabotage, I suggest that you give this book to your relative so that he or she can better understand the compulsive overeater's situation. Or you can try explaining matter-of-factly what is going on.

"My husband was becoming uptight over my partner's frequent phone calls and the time I spent at meetings," says Jennifer. "I could feel his resentment, and when he suggested one night that I have some dessert, I explained to him that all of these disruptions were really necessary for me to finally conquer my overeating problem.

"I told him that the calling-in system, as inconvenient as it may seem at times, was a way that I had finally learned to manage my overeating. I said that I would eventually be adjusting to a less hectic schedule, but just because I was spending time with my partner didn't mean I loved him any less.

"I told him something my partner had said—that by learning to love and respect myself more through this program, I would be able to express my love more fully to my husband."

Talk with your partner today about how you can best approach your family members if a sabotage problem exists.

Yielding to Distractions

In my practice, I have found that some compulsive overeaters tend to become obsessed with various side issues in their quest for weight loss, and as their energies become dispersed they never really fully tackle the major problem (compulsive overeating) at hand. One woman, after successfully losing twenty-eight pounds and keeping it off, became depressed and angry about the years she had "wasted" as a polymorph and began making frequent digressions from her eating plan. Another polymorph became preoccupied with thinking about how his life would be different when his excess weight was lost and, like some unconsciously sabotaging family members, he started feeling apprehensive about the pending changes in his life.

"As I lost more weight, I became petrified about the future," recalled Ralph. "All my relationships with people and the entire world were as an overweight person, and I didn't know what it would be like to live as a thin man. I had a vague, eerie, undefinable fear of the unknown, sensing that there were many life adjustments ahead for me and my family, but not really knowing what they were. Of course, there was also a feeling of freedom and independence from a life of being twenty-five pounds overweight, but while it was exhilarating on one hand, it was also pretty scary. And I had overeating relapses whenever the fear became too much for me to handle."

For this polymorph, even though the changes were desirous and positive, they still caused anxiety.

Whatever your own particular blocks to success are, discuss them now with your partner. Raise the factors in your life that may interfere with your continuing to make this program work. With your partner's support, you can analyze, challenge, and conquer them.

EXERCISE/RELAXATION

During today's meeting, be sure you and your partner perform both the exercise and the relaxation programs. As I suggested at the last session, the exercises work best for most polymorphs at the beginning of the meeting, with the relaxation technique scheduled at the end. But no matter when you fit them into the session, both of these activities can give you a welcome respite from the day's stresses.

By now, I hope that exercising has become a comfortable part of your everyday routine, though your progress with the relaxation technique is probably still in the learning stages. Don't be discouraged if you have trouble achieving a state of complete relaxation. Everyone has difficulty the first few times they try the technique. Ironically, relaxing takes focused attention and practice. After a few more days, you and your partner will find the relaxation experience easier to attain.

Week 7

DAY 1

EVALUATING YOUR PROGRESS

To launch the discussion in today's meeting, you and your partner should ask yourselves what is going on in your life now that wasn't there last week. At the last two meetings, for example, you talked about bingeing, family sabotage, and strengthening commitments to this program. Did these dialogues affect your behavior or life situation in any way?

Using your best listening and supporting techniques, discuss this and other issues. Include thoughts about your progress with your respective food programs, the calling-in system, your exercising, and the relaxation technique.

"I've been doing extraordinarily well with this program," Dorothy told her partner. "And I admit now that I was getting a little lax occasionally. Sometimes I would eat something without telling you. I realize now that it could have been the first step to bigger problems. Since the discussion last week, I've been really diligent in abiding by my commitments. And I feel better because of it."

For Dorothy, as with many other polymorphs, the progress she had experienced week after week had made her overconfident, feeling that even if problems did occur she could—and should—manage them alone. But the eating-behavior changes in this no-diet program are dependent upon the mutual-support systems, and are gradual and cumulative. Success builds upon success—and takes time.

So for the *full* ten weeks, you must remain thoroughly attentive to this program. For maximum effectiveness, *every* process must be carried out and fully experienced. No matter how delighted you are now by your loss of weight and your improved state of well-being, don't allow yourself to relax. Major setbacks can occur unless you maintain a healthy vigilance against subtle or obvious problems. The final few weeks are just as important as the ones that have already passed.

The most important ingredient to your success is still a partner willing to listen, support, and guide. If, for example, you are having difficulty controlling your midday snacking, your friend's job is to help you understand and solve that problem, with questions such as: "I know you didn't have this trouble two weeks ago. Are there any changes in your relationship with the people around you that might be triggering this behavior?" or "Whenever you feel the urge to reach for a snack, let's talk about it. Please call me."

Cooperation and support are crucial.

HOW GOOD ARE YOU?

An extremely valuable outgrowth of this program is a change in your self-perception. Not only will your loss of weight make you feel more positive about yourself, but so will your enriching relationship with your partner.

Your self-esteem has probably already increased significantly since the program began, although it still may not have improved as much as it eventually will. I now want you to participate in an exercise intended to help you understand just how you perceive yourself today. Sit opposite your partner and then, taking turns, tell him one good quality that you possess.

It can pertain to your achievements, intelligence, interests, appearance, or relationships, and it must be concrete and truthful:

> "I'm a responsible person."
>
> "I'm good at my work."
>
> "I'm sensitive to my parents' needs."
>
> "I keep our home running smoothly."
>
> "I'm a good friend."
>
> "I'm raising three children extremely well."
>
> "I'm a good tennis player."
>
> "I'm a great cook."

The number of favorable attributes each of you possesses is endless, but some polymorphs have difficulty specifying even one or two good qualities about themselves. As I've mentioned earlier, the compulsive overeater is often so unhappy with his body shape, and so preoccupied with how he looks, that he forgets about the other qualities that make up his personality. Thus, when asked to list his positive attributes, he has considerable trouble doing so. Ironically, most people—polymorphs or not—find it easier to think of negative rather than positive qualities about themselves.

As you and your partner continue this exercise, alternating positive statements about yourselves, you may honestly feel that you have said all there is to say. Force yourselves to continue. Make your lists longer and longer.

Even if this exercise seems difficult, you are almost certainly doing better with it than you would have six weeks ago. In the process of learning to successfully manage your polymorphism, your overall self-esteem necessarily increases as well. So by this point in the program, people invariably feel more capable, effective, and accomplished, and this exercise will reflect those changes.

After several minutes of this list-making, switch tactics: now state some positive qualities about *each other.* Tell your partner some good things about himself, and he, in turn, will do the same with you. Continue this process until you have both exhausted your praise for one another.

As you'll notice, the second part of the exercise is much easier than the first. You can more easily perceive your friend's virtues than your own. When you can think of something to say in self-praise, you may overqualify it, diminishing its importance: "I'm a *reasonably* trustworthy person"; "I have a *pretty* good sense of humor"; "I'm *not bad* as a parent."

The locus of control for reforming a poor self-image lies within each individual. Because of the issues that you've explored in this program thus far, you're probably feeling better about yourself. But there's still more room for improvement.

For the next thirty minutes, you and your partner should explore your respective self-images. The exercise above has given you a good springboard for discussion; it reflects how *you* feel about yourself today and also your positive qualities, which you may be ignoring but which your partner is very aware of. In sharing your thoughts on this issue of self-image, you can use the following questions as guidelines:

Judging by the positive qualities you listed earlier, has your self-esteem improved in the past seven weeks? If so, to what do you attribute this improvement?

Was your self-image of several weeks ago a fair appraisal of yourself?

How do you think losing weight has affected your self-esteem? Do you now feel better about any aspects of yourself other than your weight?

Were the positive qualities your partner mentioned

about you valid? If so, why do you think you didn't list them yourself?

How do you want to be perceived?

Do you sense your life changing, and, if so, do you anticipate developing even more positive feelings about yourself? How do you think this will affect your future?

In this discussion, a patient named Carl recognized how dramatically his self-image had improved. "At the beginning of this program," said Carl, "I wasn't getting what I wanted out of life, but I also didn't think I deserved to. I hardly had any feelings of self-worth, and that made me inhibited around other people.

"But the thing that started changing my self-image was the recognition that I was really helping my partner. He was losing a lot of weight, and he gave my support most of the credit. Several times, he thanked me for changing his life."

Carl's self-esteem gradually improved and, as it did, he realized how unfair his attitude toward himself had once been. "I started feeling worthwhile," he said. "If I could help my partner, I felt there were a lot of other things in life I could do, too."

While physically losing weight will help elevate your self-esteem, the entire process of support and close communication in this program will play an even more significant role. It's important, then, for you to demonstrate as much interest and concern for your partner as possible, without losing sight of your own program. Occasionally, a polymorph will become so involved in his partner's problems that he will abandon his own, thereby suffering some major regressions. You and your friend should make certain that neither of you, while offering each other support, is ignoring your own recovery from compulsive overeating.

EXERCISE/RELAXATION

Before you and your partner close today's meeting, be certain that you exercise and relax together. After your discussion of self-image, these activities will be particularly meaningful, since they have contributed significantly to the improved way you feel about yourself. They have permitted you to assume some control over your body, after perhaps years of believing that your physical self has existed outside your realm of influence. Enjoy these activities not only for the immediate pleasure they provide, but for the long-term benefits you can derive from them.

DAY 2

EVALUATING YOUR PROGRESS

At about this stage of the ten-week plan, some polymorphs start becoming anxious to weigh themselves again. Two weeks have passed since you last stepped on the scale, and that may seem like an eternity when curiosity is gnawing at you. If this is occurring with either you or your partner, make it a topic of your discussion here, along with any other relevant subjects you'd like to raise.

Let me advise you again *not* to yield to the temptation to weigh yourself now. As I've mentioned before, it is misleading and self-defeating to become dependent on the scale. If you weigh yourself constantly and are disappointed by the results on any particular day, you might decide in your frustration to abandon the program. Even if the reading on the scale thoroughly delights you, you might react by celebrating your ability to control your food intake by overeating.

Your weight on any particular day is unimportant. This

is a gradual, long-term weight-control program. By following the plan, you and your partner *will* lose weight permanently over the long haul.

This opening dialogue about your progress with the program, including the eating plan and the calling-in system, need not last more than a few minutes, or it can take up a large part of today's session. You be the judge. Offer the support that's necessary to help the two of you follow a sensible eating program. As you now know, emotional nourishment from your partner is more satisfying than food.

ASSERTIVE BEHAVIOR

When a family member, friend, or employer makes an unreasonable demand, do you have difficulty saying no?

Do you sometimes buy things that you don't even want because you're afraid to say no?

Do you feel people tend to exploit you or push you around?

Is it easier for you to smother your feelings than to openly express anger?

Do scenes like this sound familiar? Do you have difficulty telling people exactly what you want and getting them to comply with your desires? Assertiveness is directly related to self-esteem, which you and your partner have already talked about many times throughout this program. If you feel unworthy, it's hard for you to take a stand for anything. When offered a slice of cake at a dinner party, a passive polymorph might say, "Well . . . gee, if you insist . . . ah . . . okay, I'll take a piece." But the assertive polymorph would reply, "The cake looks delicious, but I'm sticking to a food plan and I really don't want any cake tonight. Thanks."

People tend to get talked into doing things they'd rather not do. And while being coerced into, say, running errands for others may seem unrelated to your compulsive overeating, it may be indicative of an inability to take control of your life and put your eating habits, and many other things, in order.

A few patients have told me that if they become assertive, they fear hurting and offending others. As one man said, "People have made fun of my obesity all my life. I know what it's like to feel abused and stepped on, and I don't want to do that to anyone else."

But when you express yourself assertively in the proper manner, no one needs to be hurt. In fact, assertive behavior is often defined as "self-expression without abusing the rights of others." When people sense you're being honest with them, it's unlikely that they will feel offended. And in the process you'll feel better about yourself, with less of the frustration and anger that drives polymorphs toward food.

"I always sensed that the people around me were manipulating me," recalls Sara. "Then, because of this ten-week program, I started cooking differently for my family, getting rid of all the foods that used to tempt me. When I eliminated sweets from our diet, my family would say things like, 'If you loved us, you'd spend some of your time baking cakes for us again,' or 'If you were a good mother and wife, you'd have some ice cream in the house for the people who wanted it.'

"I eventually learned to counter that manipulation through self-assertiveness. Often, all I'd do was separate the message into its parts and assert myself by using the word 'and.' I remember telling the family, 'I do love you, *and* I'm not going to bake cakes anymore. You can buy a slice at the coffee shop.' And I told my husband, 'I am a good wife, *and* I don't want ice cream in the house where it might cause me problems.' I found out that I didn't have to be manipulated. I began feeling better about myself as a person and about the people I love."

I'd now like you and your partner to discuss your own self-assertiveness. Do you, for example, have trouble saying no to people? Do you find that even when you turn down the requests of others, you do so apologetically?

One polymorph recognized that she often said things like "I feel just terrible telling you this, but I've decided not to volunteer at the school carnival next weekend." She was immediately placing herself on the defensive by assuming an apologetic stance. It may have been appropriate to offer a short explanation for refusing the request ("I have other commitments on Saturday"), but burdening herself with guilt was entirely unnecessary.

Here are some other specific questions you and your partner can ask one another to evaluate your own self-assertive behavior:

Are you as self-confident as you'd like to be?

Do you often feel powerless to influence a particular situation?

Are you shyer than you'd like to be?

Can you tell your spouse, friends, children, or boss exactly what's on your mind?

Can you express anger to the proper person at the moment you feel it, or do you release your aggressions through eating?

Do you say yes to almost anything that is asked of you?

To get along in the world, do you sometimes feel like you have to please others—possibly to your own detriment?

Do you fear losing the love of others if you express yourself honestly?

To improve your own assertiveness, there are many specific techniques that you can integrate into your life. Dr.

Manuel J. Smith, a psychologist, described several of them in his book, *When I Say No, I Feel Guilty,* and I recommend that my own patients integrate them into their lives. They include:

Broken Record

This technique requires that you repeatedly and calmly communicate what you want despite anyone's attempts to side-track or sway you. Even when someone won't take no for an answer, don't budge from your original statement—"I'm not going to change my shopping list to include those fattening foods"—and say it again and again, in a relaxed, unexcited tone of voice. It's not being stubborn, it's simply clearly repeating a message until it's received.

In this type of situation, being persistent is sometimes not easy. The other person may try to distract you with his own "logical" reasons why you should conform to his wishes. Using the broken-record technique, your task is to communicate a message and achieve a desired result. Do not respond to side issues until you have achieved your goal. Be conscientious, and say repeatedly, "I've decided what my own best interests are, and they require that I follow this plan exactly."

Fogging

In this skill, you acknowledge that the other person's statement may have validity, but you still do not choose to agree with it. In a sense, you may agree in principle with the other person—you're not trying to change his mind, you just don't happen to accept it yourself. Typically, you might paraphrase his statement or request, but avoid embracing it as the truth for you. For instance:

> "I can understand exactly why you feel the way you do. That's an interesting viewpoint."

"Yes, some people have lost weight on that fad diet. But I've found a different kind of program that's working well for me."

"I hear that you'd like some help with the dishes tonight. But I'm very tired, and my half of the job will have to wait until morning."

Workable Compromise

When your self-respect is not endangered by doing so, you may wish to settle a conflict in a manner acceptable to both parties. This technique is often used as a practical solution to a problem that otherwise seems unresolvable. The other person, however, must be willing to listen openly to your point of view.

Let's assume, for example, that your partner wanted to hurry through this discussion to a later segment of the program, but you were interested in learning more about this issue. You might tell him, "Why don't we finish this discussion on assertiveness, and then we'll get into the subjects you're most interested in?" Or if your partner resists joining you in some weekend walks together, you can suggest, "Let's try it for two weekends. If you still don't like it, then we'll try something else."

Negative Assertion

With this technique, while accepting valid criticism you forcefully and comfortably examine your own negative qualities. This allows you to quiet the other person's criticism while simultaneously judging yourself rather than allowing him to do so. You might, for instance, simply tell a criticizing relative, "There is no doubt I have a serious weight problem that I need to do something about. I don't like being overweight." Or if you're late for one of your meetings with your partner, you can tell him, "That was so wrong of me to forget the starting time," instead of reacting with anger of your own, like "What do you mean? You mess things up a lot, too."

Self-Disclosure

This skill requires you to assertively reveal your thoughts about your own personality, lifestyle, and behavior. In the process, you not only improve communication but also surprisingly *ease* your anxiety by bringing your secret thoughts about yourself out into the open where they can no longer gnaw at you out of conscious awareness. Statements such as "I feel anxious, confused, and/or fearful," which you usually avoid, are the very ones that validate your strength. (It takes a powerful person to openly share that he or she *feels* weak.) This kind of openness will also allow the people you're communicating with the space to share their own insecurities. *It is one of the best techniques for opening up communication.*

For example, if family members criticize the intensity of your current effort at losing weight because they feel they have less of your time, you can honestly respond with "I was copping out with all the diets I've tried in the past and I still feel confused and anxious about my new program. But I'm starting to learn about myself now, and losing weight in the process. Please be patient."

With your partner, familiarize yourself with these techniques and discuss ways in which they might be useful in everyday situations—with family members, friends, and coworkers. Try a psychodrama that incorporates these techniques. Also, make a commitment to actively become more assertive in your interpersonal relationships between now and your next meeting. Appropriate assertiveness can make a positive difference in how you feel about yourself and those around you.

If you'd like a more detailed explanation of assertive techniques, I suggest you read *When I Say No, I Feel Guilty* by Dr. Manuel J. Smith.

EXERCISE/RELAXATION

In today's meeting, you should both exercise with your partner and practice the relaxation technique with him. Relaxation techniques are an integral part of most assertiveness-training courses. Experts agree that acting assertively is easier when you are free of tension or nervousness.

By now, exercising should be part of your life. A regular, moderate exercise regimen will help you look better, feel better and find more enjoyment in life.

In the intervening days between now and your next meeting, I want you to think about how dramatically your attitudes and eating habits have changed in the last seven weeks. You have achieved a lot, including a gradual but continuous loss of weight. You have probably already accomplished more here than with any diet you've ever been on. The remainder of the program will help determine just how permanent your weight loss will be. Make a strong commitment to proceed faithfully through the final three weeks with your partner.

Week 8

DAY 1

EVALUATING YOUR PROGRESS

For the next few minutes, you and your partner should share your thoughts on how the program is proceeding for each of you. If you are still having frequent, or even just occasional, problems, it's a good idea to keep a list during the week of the difficulties you're facing and bring it to the meeting. With the list in hand, you won't forget to raise any of the issues that may have surfaced in recent days and which haven't already been discussed during your daily phone calls.

Be certain to continue telephoning your daily menu to your partner. This system will make you thoroughly aware of when and what you are eating, which can deter you from consuming food on a whim, without really being aware of it.

"For years, I used to eat a few handfuls of wheat crackers every evening while reading the newspaper," says Diane. "But I cut them out of my eating plan when I started this program, and I know it's made a difference. Even though this no-diet approach doesn't emphasize calorie counting, I still figured that I had lost—and kept off—a few pounds just by making this relatively minor change in my eating. And the calling-in system helped me maintain it."

PRACTICING ASSERTIVENESS TRAINING

At the last meeting, you were introduced to the concept of assertiveness training. In essence, assertiveness is an affirmation of the self. It is a sensible stance assumed by individuals who rightfully believe that their thoughts and feelings matter. An assertive person can express his anger and his happiness, his love and his dissatisfaction.

Nonassertive people rarely voice their feelings and needs, and consequently are often dominated by others. In turn, they may overeat to deal with their frustrations. Thus, if you can improve your assertiveness, you can resolve some of the anxiety that may be triggering your overeating.

The best way to prepare yourself for a more assertive lifestyle is for you and your partner to conduct a "behavior rehearsal," in which each of you acts out the assertiveness you plan to adopt in an upcoming real-life situation. This activity is similar to the psychodrama that was introduced to you in Week 4. The two of you will role-play—that is, simulate reality without the fears and perils of an actual confrontation.

Think of a situation you want to work on. Are you involved in a relationship with a spouse, a child, or a parent that may be contributing to your polymorphism and that you would like to be confronting more honestly and assertively? Select such a circumstance in your life and act it out with your partner. You will play yourself, and your partner will portray the other party to your new behavior. Refer back to Week 7 to refresh your memory on the specific techniques to use in assertiveness training—techniques like fogging, negative assertion, and workable compromise.

During this session, Beth decided to rehearse a discussion she wanted to have with her boyfriend, Tom, who was starting to feel threatened by her involvement in her no-diet program. With her partner, Rose, assuming the role of her boyfriend, Beth had a behavioral-rehearsal discussion with "Tom." Because Beth had talked so much about Tom's feelings during their meetings, Rose had little difficulty playing Tom's role. Their behavioral rehearsal included the following exchange:

ROSE (AS TOM): "There are too many things happening with this program. There are phone calls at any time and those long meetings with Rose. The time you spend with her could be spent with me instead."

BETH: "I really feel I'm doing the right thing and I understand how you feel, but it's been difficult for me to lose weight in the past. Even when I've lost it, I've always gained it back. But this program is working, and Rose's support is one of the reasons why."

ROSE (AS TOM): "But wouldn't you rather be with me? I bet we could find a diet you can go on that wouldn't take so much of your time."

BETH: "I appreciate your viewpoint, but I need this program now. That doesn't mean I don't need you, too. But for me to feel good about myself, I've got to lose this weight once and for all. I'd like to talk about this more with you so that you'll know exactly how I feel."

In this exchange, Beth expressed her feelings honestly and directly. She made concrete statements about her needs and desires, and also declared a willingness to spend time making her viewpoints even better understood.

In addition to this behavioral rehearsal, practice assertive behavior in the upcoming days. It's okay to say no when someone asks you for something that's unfair or impractical. After all, receiving someone's love should not be conditioned on what you do for him or her, but rather on who you are.

EXERCISE/RELAXATION

During today's meeting, be sure to exercise with your partner and to practice your relaxation technique together. Some polymorphs find the relaxation technique so therapeutic that they practice it two or three times a day to turn off inner tension and reassert control over their bodies. And, of course, any additional physical exercise you can add to your day will make you feel even better about yourself and your body.

DAY 2

EVALUATING YOUR PROGRESS

If you have any thoughts and feelings about the no-diet program, this is the time to discuss them with your partner. For example, have there been any emotional disruptions in your life recently that have triggered a midnight binge or provoked thoughts of one? Now is the time to talk about it. In the process, you will reaffirm just how nourishing your partner's support can be.

Discuss any other relevant topics as well. Perhaps you are beginning to feel some resistance to attending these meetings. "I'm losing weight and can feel the momentum building," said one patient, "and I think I can handle things on my own from now on." As I've said before, don't submit to such temptation. Despite the dramatic progress you may have experienced, your partner's support can help make your new attitudes an even more significant part of your life.

Katy, a high-school teacher, recently explained the important role that she and her partner had played in one another's lives. "Until I started on this program, my whole life was food. When I wasn't eating, I was *thinking* about eating. Or

I was reading about fad diets in women's magazines. I was terribly unhappy with my life, but I didn't feel capable of changing it.

"My partner, though, gave me the encouragement I had never had before. When I finally felt good about the way this program was going, she was there to share it with me. And, of course, I did the same for her. When she got depressed during the difficult times, I encouraged her to stick with it. We called each other at all hours of the day and night—at home, in restaurants, at parties, everywhere. There was never a time when we were unavailable. And when we helped each other, it gave us a psychological boost that kept us going for days."

Your partner is more critical to this program than when or what you eat.

HOW YOU SEE YOURSELF—THEN AND NOW

This unique approach to weight loss is designed to guide you and your partner through a transformation. As you change your eating habits, you will not only lose weight permanently but you will also alter the way you feel about yourself.

In the next thirty to forty-five minutes, I'd like you and your partner to have another discussion about your self-image—specifically, how did you see yourself in the first week of this program, and how do you see yourself now?

As I have mentioned repeatedly, negative body image is a serious problem for many compulsive overeaters. They have internalized society's negative feelings about obesity, integrating them into their own belief system. And the anxiety created by this poor self-esteem can cause overeating.

One polymorph, for example, was very successful in business. But because of his low self-esteem, which grew out of his overweight problem, he didn't feel worthy of the success he was achieving. He had become convinced that he would never make anything of himself, so he presumed that each major step forward in his career was merely a stroke of luck, and that he didn't actually deserve it. Inevitably, he would binge, gaining even more pounds, as an unconscious way of proving to the world that he really wasn't as worthy as his success seemed to indicate.

In one extreme case, a polymorph had been told by her father since early childhood that she was worthless; later in life, she became a battered wife. But she never complained about the beatings, either to her spouse or to the police. Due to her low self-esteem, she believed that she "deserved" this physical abuse, just as she "deserved" the obesity she was inflicting upon herself. Although her father had died many years earlier, she had incorporated his opinions into her belief system, resulting in such self-hatred that she believed herself undeserving of any kindness.

Even if you had low self-esteem or a negative body image when you entered this program, by now you've begun to experience the *real* you. You've examined yourself as you actually are, not as you have been programed to see yourself. Gradually, you've started to take control of your life and to feel better about yourself. And there has probably been a positive change in the way the people in your environment feel about you, too.

Take as much time as you need now to share with your partner the ways in which your self-image has evolved in recent weeks. Also ask yourselves about the feedback you've gotten from others. Have they noticed changes in your attitudes or behavior, in addition to your weight loss? Share all the positive things that have happened in your life in recent weeks.

Finally, to give you plenty of time to prepare for your first meeting in Week 10, I want you to process the pictures you took during the first week of this program. We'll be using those pictures in the tenth week as still another look at the "old" in contrast to the "new" you.

EXERCISE/RELAXATION

During today's session, be sure you and your partner perform the physical exercise regimen and the relaxation technique. Once again, I suggest exercising at the beginning of the meeting, and relaxing at the end. If you've been performing the relaxation technique conscientiously, you can probably bring your body to a state of total relaxation much faster than you could the first few times you tried it. You're gaining more command over your body and allowing yourself to enjoy the experience of being in control.

Week 9

DAY 1

Throughout this program, you have had the opportunity to create an unusual, intimate relationship with your partner. Each of you has relied on the other for constant support in the last eight weeks, and in the process of assisting one another, you have formed a friendship that may well be closer and warmer than any you've had.

In addition to your partner, there will be another, different kind of support system that you can also depend upon soon—your closest family members. In the weeks and months ahead, they can help you maintain or continue your weight loss by supporting you in your control of the polymorph syndrome. You won't necessarily be discussing sensitive weight-related issues with the same degree of intimacy that you have established with your partner (you may do so if you wish, of course). Still, family members can commit themselves to your well-being by offering understanding, cooperation, and encouragement. With their positive involvement in the future, your weight loss will be permanent.

There are several ways you can draw your family members into your weight-loss regimen this week. Earlier in the program, I suggested that you respond to their inquiries or insecurities about this ten-week plan by giving them this book to read or merely by answering their questions matter-of-factly. Certainly, giving them this book to read now would be very productive. But I want you to do even more. To ensure their active support and encouragement of you, please invite them to your next meeting. For that next session, you and your partner will ask those persons closest to each of you—spouses, children, parents, lovers, roommates—to join you.

Some polymorphs feel apprehensive about inviting their family's participation. These loved ones may have expressed some skepticism or impatience about this program. You may be afraid that they will dominate that session with criticism. Some polymorphs even feel that involving other people, even if they are family members, will disrupt or intrude upon the special relationship they have developed with their partner.

For the next few minutes, discuss with your partner any anxieties you each may have about setting up a family session. What do you believe might happen? What are the criticisms, if any, that you anticipate? What do you imagine your response would be? What positive side effects might there be to the meeting as well?

In my experience with polymorphs, most of their concerns at this time prove to be largely unfounded and, more important, seem much less threatening once they are out in the open. Your own worst fears are probably exaggerated far beyond what really will happen.

To encourage family members to attend this meeting, be willing to adjust the time and day of that session for the convenience of everyone involved. Discuss with your partner the best time and place for that meeting, and then verify it with each other in a day or two to confirm the arrangements.

Some family members may resist your invitation to attend the meeting. In my experience, the reason for this resistance is fear of the unknown ("What are the two of you going to do—tell me everything I've been doing wrong all these years that's caused you to become fat?"). I suggest that you positively and directly express your desire for their attendance and your need for their support. Tell them that for the program to continue successfully, you will need their help. And for them to help you fully, they should be completely aware of the impact this program has had on you and the new role they will be playing in your life.

EVALUATING YOUR PROGRESS

As you normally do in the early stages of each meeting, you and your partner should talk now about any issues that have arisen in the past few days that may be relevant to the program. One polymorph, delighted with her successful weight reduction, chose to spend this time talking about how the daily menu planning and phone conversations with her partner had finally evolved from the most difficult to the most helpful aspect of this program.

"Until I started this no-diet plan, I was used to 'feast or famine' living," she told me later. "I would crash diet, then binge, and then diet again. But when I made a real commitment to this calling-in plan, I started eating sensibly, and never really felt like I was depriving myself. That's when I really began losing weight."

DISCUSSING YOUR ASSERTIVENESS

One of the purposes of this program has been to increase your self-confidence and your sense of self-worth. The assertiveness techniques that I introduced you to can play an important role in this process, by allowing you to deal effectively with the people around you. I hope you have started incorporating them into your daily life by now. Spend a few minutes here sharing your experiences with your partner.

Continue to incorporate assertiveness techniques into your interactions with other people. They will make a significant difference in your self-perception.

EXERCISE/RELAXATION

As part of today's meeting, be sure to both exercise and relax. By now, I hope you have also discovered other ways to incorporate physical activity into your daily life aside from your regular exercise schedule. A recent study revealed, for example, that if you were to climb the stairs to your fourth-floor office four times a day, this action alone would cause you to lose nine pounds a year. If you continue daily exercising indefinitely, you can count on achieving steady, continuous weight maintenance or reduction, depending on your caloric intake.

DAY 2

MEETING WITH THE FAMILIES

This meeting is devoted to an open-ended discussion with the spouses, children, parents, lovers, and/or roommates you and your partner have invited. All of the participants should sit together in a group and, in a casual, unstructured manner, discuss some of the issues that each of you would like to raise.

There are some general guidelines I would like all of you to follow in this meeting, which are the communication techniques that I described in Chapter 4. You may want to refer to them to refresh your memory. Particularly keep in mind that your job is not to judge, give advice, or provide the "definitive solutions" to everyone's dilemmas. While you can tell others in the group what your own best interests may be, don't form conclusions for them about their own needs and desires. Avoid words like "should" and "ought."

I also suggest that when a sensitive subject is being discussed, such as the issue of sabotage, *your partner lead the conversation with your family and you do the same with his family.* You and your partner have learned a lot about one another in the past few weeks, and it may be easier for him to raise certain issues involving those closest to you. He may be able to launch discussions on certain topics in a less tension-inducing way than you could.

I recall a young woman named Lorraine who believed that for years her mother had intentionally spoiled every attempt the young woman had made at losing weight. Her mother, said Lorraine, was convinced that if her daughter became thin, and was thus attractive to men, she would lose her. "As much as I asked her not to," recalls Lorraine, "Mom always had candy and other problem foods around the house. I'd get derailed from a diet just a few days after I started it."

Lorraine had raised this issue with her mother several times over the years, with little success. So in this family session, Lorraine felt that her partner might be better able to raise the issue objectively and present an unbiased point of view of the situation. Thus, her partner talked about the subject of sabotage and how it is unconsciously practiced by family members who really have no intention of hurting their loved ones. The partner even asked Lorraine's mother some relevant questions ("Do you think the choices of food around the house could pose a dangerous temptation for Lorraine when she is trying to change her eating habits?"; "Would she perhaps have an easier time of it if those foods weren't there?"; "What if Lorraine were to be thin—do you think her relationship with you would change?").

As Lorraine's mother heard the subject discussed from an impartial vantage point, she listened intently. She responded to questions, and for the first time, she was truly able to understand her daughter. That relationship began to change, and Lorraine's mother started to become more supportive of her daughter's feelings.

Lorraine's mother had not been acting out of malice. If your own family members attempt to keep you dependent, it's not because they want to hurt you. They are merely fearful of change.

You may say to your mother, spouse, or other family member, "I know you're trying to help me, and I know it's hard not to make those comments. But please allow *me* to monitor my behavior rather than you. I love you, and I know you love me, so please help support me in controlling my compulsive overeating. It would also help me if certain foods weren't so available or conspicuous in the household."

A good starting point for this meeting is for you and your partner to talk about the important role you want your family members to start playing. Tell them that, beginning today, you are enlisting their support in helping you make your weight loss permanent. They can be a major influence on your frame of mind and your eating behavior. Let them know that you need their love, warmth, and encouragement.

Early in the meeting, you and your partner can also discuss what has transpired between the two of you during the last nine weeks. If you haven't talked with your family much about the program in the last two months, even the concept of polymorphism may be as foreign to them as it once was to you, and it's important for them to understand it. Discuss the dynamics behind your compulsive overeating as you comprehend them. Explain the no-diet program and what you're willing to discuss about your relationships with the people in your past and present. Ask your loved ones whether they have any questions or concerns.

In the opening minutes of the family meeting, one or more family members will sometimes complain that they can't talk openly in front of so many people. Encourage them to please remain flexible and open-minded, and see if their feelings change. Most people's apprehensions are gradually eased, particularly once they recognize that everyone is simply trying to help one another.

Despite their fears to the contrary, most polymorphs report that they rarely encounter real anger or conflict from their family members. But if you do, try applying some of the assertiveness techniques you have learned to defuse the conflict. For instance, try fogging, in which you concede that your family members' opinions may make sense for them but that you have different thoughts and feelings ("I see why you've been upset by some of the things I've done, but they've helped me lose weight, which I hope you're happy about"). Or you might apply the workable-compromise technique ("I'd appreciate any time you can spend with me on the no-diet program; is there something I can do for you to reciprocate?").

The most important goal of this meeting is to obtain a commitment from your family to support you in the months ahead. In the process, as the dialogue among all participants becomes more free-flowing and uninhibited, the meeting may evolve into one of the most important of this ten-week program. Let it take its own course and run as long as necessary for everyone to feel they have shared, learned, and come to an understanding as to their future commitments to one another.

Next week, you and your partner will discuss your reactions to this meeting and what has happened in the ensuing days in your family relationships.

Week 10

DAY 1

In the last two meetings of the final week of the program, you and your partner will be reviewing and evaluating what you have learned, how much you've achieved, and your future expectations. You've come a long way, lost weight, and more important, acquired the tools you need to keep it off forever Whenever someone compliments you on your new attitudes toward life or on how good you look, you should justifiably feel a tremendous sense of accomplishment. Before this week is over, you and your partner will solidify your commitment to maintain your weight loss for the rest of your life.

THE FAMILY MEETING REVIEWED

Devote the beginning of today's session to a discussion of the family meeting you held last time. For some polymorphs, that session became a landmark in their lives, a time in which they opened up communication channels with their spouse, children, or parents that had never been there before. At that meeting, you may also have touched on areas of misunderstanding that you can now work on openly. You may have successfully dealt with major issues like unconscious sabotage, which was threatening to undermine your success with this program.

Discuss with your partner your respective reactions to the family meeting and what has happened since then. In the days immediately following the family gathering, one man told his wife, "I never realized until that get-together how much pain you've felt being overweight. If I had known, I would have offered you my support long ago. I want to help now in any way I can."

At this follow-up meeting, one woman told her partner that her children had agreed to try to stop their unconscious sabotage. "They came to me the day after the family meeting and told me to point out their sabotage to them whenever it happens," she said. "They thought they were being loving by bringing me something to eat. They had no idea that they had been working against me, not with me."

If your family meeting was successful, and particularly if you feel there are still more issues to be discussed and resolved (which there often are), you and your partner may decide to schedule another session with your families this week. A continuing dialogue with those closest to you can only improve your chances of permanent weight loss as you begin relying on them for encouragement and understanding during times of crisis when you feel tempted to binge.

So talk to your partner now about having a second family meeting if you wish to strengthen everyone's commitment to help one another. Some families find that the second meeting is even more worthwhile than the first. Everyone is usually relaxed from the start this time, without any of the fears they may have brought with them the previous week. And because they now feel a part of the program, they're usually eager to discuss the contribution *they* can make to help this program work permanently.

EVALUATING YOUR PROGRESS

Even without a scale, I'm sure you're aware of the success you've had with this program. Most polymorphs report that they've been complimented by friends on how good they look, and that they are aware of more energy and more self-confidence. Today, you and your partner will weigh and measure yourselves and record the results on the chart you began in Week 1. I think you'll be pleased with the results. The new eating habits you've learned in this program are the tools that can keep your weight off for good and permit you to lose even more if you desire. In addition to your new attitudes toward eating and your consequent weight loss from this program, you've also formed a valuable friendship and more positive feelings about yourself—benefits every bit as important as the lost pounds, if not more so.

In the future, I hope you will continue to weigh yourself only once a month. That way, you'll obtain a more realistic picture of how you're doing and not be discouraged because you don't lose a fraction of a pound on a particular day.

To further solidify your success with this program, I would now like the two of you to take still another step forward. Bring out the snapshots you have brought with you today, and discuss with your partner who and what you see. Of course, you're still the same person. But in those photos, do you also see someone different, not only heavier, but also someone who thinks and feels differently than you do now?

In a sense, you are *not* who you were when this program began. You have come to think of yourself as a more worthwhile person, one who has many positive attributes that you once probably ignored. Spend a few minutes now discussing the changes in yourself and how you feel about them.

Even though you feel better about yourself now than you did during the first week of the program, many polymorphs also experience a sense of loss after successfully losing weight.

1. *You've lost part of your body.* As a thinner person, you no longer have the extra layer of fat that you may once have used subconsciously to protect yourself from the outside world. Most polymorphs are surprised to feel a temporary sense of emptiness because of this. But this sensation disappears once they and their partners clearly become aware that they are now prepared to deal with the world effectively and no longer need this artificial barrier.

2. *You've lost aspects of your old personality.* Shedding excess weight may also change some of your personality characteristics. You new sense of self-confidence can result in more appropriate and adaptive actions, letting go of old behaviors ranging from false gregariousness or even a pushy personality to extreme shyness.

3. *You've lost your "best" friend.* For years, food was the constant companion you relied upon for comfort. Although it was destructive, such an intimate relationship is difficult to abandon fully. Fortunately, you've developed a real relationship with your partner and a strengthened bond with your family, which will fill the void that your withdrawal from overeating has left, providing more nourishment than food ever did. In the future, you will find that the capacity you've developed for warm relationships will extend to others in your life.

As unusual as these "losses" may seem at first glance, they are very real for some polymorphs. True, you are probably glad to say goodbye to those negative aspects of your life. But even so, they have been familiar parts of your existence for years, and thus the process of transformation is sometimes difficult. Fortunately, any sense of loss is usually short-lived. Even though you are saying goodbye to the "old" you, you are also welcoming a new self. And I'm sure you are proud of how far you've come.

During this meeting, it will also be useful for you and your partner to talk about your food plan and the role it will play in the future. After this tenth week ends, you must continue planning your menus in advance and calling your partner.

Even so, in the weeks and months ahead, you might still have occasional bingeing episodes or find yourself eating foods you hadn't planned to. Reassure yourself that you don't have to be perfect. If slips happen, you now have your partner and an awareness of and a method of dealing with the skills to evaluate what is going on in your life and the effect it may be having on your eating. You are now capable of eliminating the cause of your self-destructive behavior.

If you're having trouble, remember what you learned while keeping the Food Diary; ask yourself what mood, event, or activity may be causing the problem. Most important, talk to your partner or to a family member if cravings occur. You now have a larger support system than ever before.

EXERCISE/RELAXATION

During today's session, be sure to engage in your exercises and the relaxation technique. In the weeks ahead, plan to continue both as a part of your daily routine. One woman, for instance, told me that she exercises each morning and night while watching television, which not only benefits her body in its own right, but also keeps her from eating while she watches TV.

In addition to your regular exercise program, keep thinking of other types of physical activities that you can incorporate into your life. One man canceled his subscription to his daily newspaper and started walking six blocks each morning to buy his paper at the supermarket. A woman bought a puppy and took it for long walks every evening. Another polymorph bought bicycles for herself and her husband, and they ride them almost every weekend.

In the future, you should continue to use the relaxation technique. Each time you practice it, you will be gaining more control over your body—and your polymorphism.

DAY 2

THE LAST FEW POUNDS

In my experience, most polymorphs are able to lose their excess weight successfully except for the last few pounds.

This phenomenon is baffling to many overeaters. After all, they've lost so much already; why can't they just lose a few more pounds? After you understand the dynamics of this obstacle, you will finally be able to overcome it.

Consider the fact that for years you may have fantasized about being at your ideal weight and the wonderful ways it would change your life. Perhaps you imagined how beautiful or handsome you'd be, how your romantic life would change, how you'd get a better job, or how your personality could finally blossom and flourish. Many of your dreams may have hinged on losing weight.

But once you've lost nearly all the weight you had hoped to lose and your life hasn't transformed as you'd fantasized it would, no longer can you explain your reality away with "Everything will be great once I'm thin." So in a sense, those last few pounds allow you still to have that fantasy and to avoid the reality of not being perfect or having the perfect job or relationship.

As you approach your "ideal" weight, many new life situations will arise. You may find yourself in competitive settings at work and in the social arena that you never faced before. People around you may react to your greater self-confidence and assertiveness with jealousy or even hostility—emotions that may never have been directed at you until now.

You must simply recognize that losing weight isn't what's going to make you happy or successful. It might make you happ*ier* or *more* successful, but it's not the magic answer. *You* are the key to your future.

If losing the last few pounds is proving difficult for you, I suggest that you approach things one day at a time. As you've discovered, you are a capable and worthwhile person. You can handle this situation the same way you've dealt with the other emotional crises you have experienced during the program—namely, share your anxieties *now* with your partner about what your life will be like when you've lost all your excess weight. You'll find that your partner may feel exactly as you do. Both of you can start dealing with these fantasies realistically. Like the weight you've already lost, you *can* conquer your anxieties about your life changes.

"My partner and I talked," recalls Dana, "and decided that despite our concerns about the future, we had already achieved a lot, and we weren't going to be deterred at this late stage. We agreed to adhere to our food plan in the future, one day at a time."

CONTINUING YOUR WEIGHT-LOSS PROGRAM

This program has asked you to explore aspects of your personality that you may have never probed before, as a path to permanently changing behavior that took years to develop. It hasn't been easy, but your successes show that it has been worth the effort. Yet, as a polymorph, in order to maintain the loss, you have to be willing to pursue a program of always scrutinizing not only what you eat but also the problems in your life that might lead to a binge—until this process becomes automatic, which it will. In order to continue reinforcing the new behavior patterns you have learned, I strongly urge you and your partner to commit yourselves to keeping this program going in some manner.

Many polymorphs decide to continue the daily calling-in system with one another and meet on a regular but less frequent basis. Better yet, others invite in another friend or two and, as a threesome or foursome, they proceed through the entire program again. But even if you'd rather limit the future meetings to only you and your partner, there's still a great deal the two you haven't shared. You'll be surprised at how much more you can learn about yourself and the polymorph syndrome the second time around. And by maintaining your relationship with your partner, and relying on your family's support as well, you will continue the support system that guarantees more weight loss or weight maintenance for the pounds already lost.

I also strongly suggest that you and your partner attend meetings of Overeaters Anonymous (OA) in your community. OA deals with many of the same issues that we have approached in this program in the last ten weeks. It is a nonprofit organization requiring no dues or fees. As you're surely now aware, the polymorph's successful weight loss is predicated on the support he gets with his problems and temptations. Your local chapter of OA is another strong link in the support network available to you.

As a recovering polymorph who has completed this experience, you now possess many positive qualities that will enhance your life in the future. Over the last few weeks, you and your partner have learned to love, respect, and care for one another and to communicate honestly. These qualities have not only helped you gain control over your polymorphism, but you can use them in every aspect of your life. You have learned to relate to people in a way that most individuals never do.

You are now a complete, more caring and intimate person. The tools you have acquired in this program will remain with you after your weight is permanently under control, *allowing* you to experience life to the fullest. Therefore, in a real sense, you are *lucky* to be a recovering polymorph.

As you leave today's session, congratulate yourselves on completing a comprehensive plan to control your polymorphism. Be proud of yourself. You deserve it.

Appendix

Food Plans

The food plans below were created by Overeaters Anonymous, a self-help organization for compulsive overeaters. They are excellent plans, and you may decide to choose one of them for this ten-week program. Before going on any food plan, however, it might be a good idea to consult your physician to determine whether you have specific needs that your diet should incorporate.

GENERAL DIRECTIONS

Food Preparation

Broil, bake, boil, roast, grill or dry-fry meats.

Read labels and avoid sugar as a main ingredient. (If sugar is listed fifth or later, the amount is negligible.)

Food Guidance

8-oz. measuring cup

Postal or kitchen scale

Measuring spoons

Spatula or butter knife for leveling

Food Abstinence Suggestions

Write down your daily food plan and call it in to your partner.

Do *not* skip meals

When in doubt, leave it out.

Sit while eating.

Slow down, relax, enjoy your meals.

Weigh yourself only once a month.

1. Basic Four[1]

Breakfast

1 serving vitamin-C-rich fruit or 4 oz. juice

2 oz. meat, fish, or meat substitute or 1 egg or 1 oz. hard cheese or 2 oz. cottage cheese

1 oz. cereal or 1 slice whole grain bread or 1 oz. wheat germ

4 oz. lowfat or skim milk

Lunch

1 cup raw or cooked vegetable or 1 fruit

4 oz. meat, fish, or meat substitute or 2 eggs or 2 oz. hard cheese or 4 oz. cottage cheese

1 oz. wheat germ or 1 slice whole-grain bread or equivalent

4 oz. lowfat or skim milk

Dinner

1 cup salad, with 1 tablespoon oil or salad dressing

---

1. See Food List I

1 cup cooked vegetable

4-6 oz. meat, fish, or meat substitute or 2 eggs or 2 oz. hard cheese or 4-6 oz. cottage cheese

4 oz. potato or rice or 1 slice whole grain bread or 1 oz. wheat germ

4 oz. lowfat or skim milk

2. Sugar and Flour Free[1]

Breakfast

2 oz. meat, fish, or meat substitute or 1 egg or 1 oz. hard cheese or 2 oz. cottage cheese

1 fruit or 4 oz. citrus fruit juice

1 oz. (2 tablespoons) wheat germ or millers bran

4 oz. lowfat or skim milk

Lunch

4 oz. meat, fish, or meat substitute or 2 eggs or 2 oz. hard cheese or 4 oz. cottage cheese

1 cup salad

3 raw vegetables or 1 cup cooked or raw vegetables

1 oz. wheat germ or millers bran (2 tablespoons)

4 oz. lowfat or skim milk

Dinner

4-6 oz. meat, fish, or meat substitute or 2 eggs or 2 oz. hard cheese or 4-6 oz. cottage cheese

1 cup salad, with 1 tablespoon oil or salad dressing[2]

1 cup cooked vegetable

1. Food List I
2. See Fats category in Food List.

1 oz. wheat germ or millers bran (2 tablespoons)

4 oz. lowfat or skim milk

3. Vegetarian[1]

Breakfast

1 vitamin C fruit or 4 oz. fruit juice

2 oz. hard cheese or 4 oz. cottage cheese or 4 oz. protein substitute or 2 oz. nuts or 1 cup lowfat plain yogurt

1 slice whole-grain bread or ½ oz. wheat germ or whole-grain cereal

4 oz. lowfat or skim milk

Lunch

2 eggs or 2 oz. hard cheese or 4 oz. cottage cheese or 4 oz. protein substitute or 2 oz. nuts or 1 cup lowfat plain yogurt

1 slice bread or ½ oz. wheat germ or whole-grain cereal

1 cup salad or green vegetable

1 fruit

4 oz. lowfat or skim milk

Dinner

4 oz. protein substitute or 2 eggs or 2-3 oz. hard cheese or 4-6 oz. cottage cheese

1 cup cooked vegetables

---

1. Food List I

2 cups salad, with 1 tablespoon dressing[2]

4 oz. lowfat or skim milk

4. Youth[1]

Breakfast

4 oz. meat, fish, or meat substitute or 2 eggs or 2 oz. hard cheese or 4 oz. cottage cheese

1 fruit

8 oz. lowfat or skim milk

1 slice whole grain bread or 1 oz. sugar-free cereal

Lunch

4 oz. meat, fish, or meat substitute or 2 eggs or 2 oz. hard cheese or 4 oz. cottage cheese

1 cup vegetable or 1 fruit   Finger salad (3 pieces raw vegetables)

8 oz. lowfat or skim milk

2 slices whole grain bread

Dinner

4-6 oz. meat or meat substitute or 2-3 oz. hard cheese or 2 eggs plus 1 oz. hard cheese or 4-6 oz. cottage cheese

1 cup vegetable

2 cups salad with 1 tablespoon dressing[2]

---

1. Food List I
2. See Fats category in Food List.

1 fruit

8 oz. lowfat or skim milk

5. Medical[1]

Note: This program is particularly designed to be shown to your doctor. Your doctor can advise you if you have any special medical dietary requirements.

Breakfast

1 serving Vitamin-C-rich fruit or juice

1 serving protein-rich food

1 serving grain product

milk

Lunch

1 serving protein-rich food

1 serving vegetable or fruit

1 or 2 servings grain product

milk

Dinner

1 serving protein-rich food

1 serving grain or grain substitute (potato, rice, etc.)

1 serving dark-green or orange vegetable salad with dressing

1 serving fruit

milk

---

1. Food List I

6. Modified Carbohydrate[1]

Breakfast

4 oz. meat, fish, or meat substitute or 2 eggs or 1 oz. hard cheese[2] or 4 oz. cottage cheese

1 Vitamin-C-rich fruit

Lunch

4 oz. meat, fish, or meat substitute or 2 eggs or 2 oz. hard cheese[2] or 4 oz. cottage cheese

1 serving vegetable

1 finger salad or fruit

Dinner

4 oz. meat, fish, or meat substitute or 2 eggs or 2 oz. hard cheese[3] or 4 oz. cottage cheese

1 serving vegetable[4]

2 cups salad with 2 tablespoons dressing[2]

7. No Refined Carbohydrates[5]

Note: With this plan, hard cheese must be eaten at least once daily, and a multivitamin is to be taken daily.

---

1. Food List I
2. See Fats category in Food List.
3. Protein may be bran, wheat germ, or whole-grain bread as defined below.
4. Once a day, ¼ cup bran or wheat germ or 1 serving whole-grain bread may be substituted for one serving vegetable.
5. Food List II

Breakfast

4 oz. meat, fish, or meat substitute or 2 pieces chicken or 2 eggs or 2 oz. hard cheese or 4 oz. cottage cheese

1 fruit

Lunch

4 oz. meat, fish, or meat substitute or 2 pieces chicken or 2 eggs or 2 oz. hard cheese or 4 oz. cottage cheese

1 serving vegetable

2 cups salad with 2 tablespoons dressing[2]

Dinner

4 oz. meat, fish, or meat substitute or 2 pieces chicken or 2 eggs or 2 oz. hard cheese or 4 oz. cottage cheese

1 serving vegetable

2 cups salad with 2 tablespoons dressing[2]

FOOD LIST I

Proteins

A. Beef

1. Lean: Veal, baby beef, chipped beef, trimmed chuck flank steak, tenderloin, plate ribs, plate skirt steak, round steak (all cuts), rump, tripe
2. Fat: Ground, ribeye, ground round, ground chuck, roasts, steaks, breast of veal

B. Lamb (lean only): Leg, rib, sirloin, loin (roast and chops), shank, shoulder

C. Pork

1. Lean: Leg (whole rump, center shank), ham (center slices)

---

2. These vegetables should be included in your menu at least 4-6 times a week.

   2. Fat: Loin (all cuts tenderloin), shoulder arm (picnic), shoulder blade, Boston butt, Canadian bacon, boiled ham, loin (back ribs), ground pork, country-style ham, deviled ham

D. Poultry

   1. Lean: Meat without skin of chicken, turkey, Cornish game hen, Guinea hen, pheasant
   2. Fat: Capon, duck, goose

E. Organ meats: Liver, heart, kidney, sweetbreads, gizzards

F. Fish

   1. Lean: Fresh, frozen, or canned cod, sole, halibut, perch, tuna, mackerel, flounder, turbot, crab, lobster, clams, oysters, scallops, shrimp, sardines (not packed in oil)
   2. Fat: salmon, herring

G. Cheese

   1. Lean: Cottage, farmer, pot cheese, part-skim ricotta
   2. Fat: Mozzarella, ricotta, cheddar, slicing cheese

H. Processed Protein (Fat): Cold cuts, frankfurters

I. Eggs (Medium fat)

J. Milk

   1. Lean: Skim buttermilk, lowfat, lowfat yogurt,[1] evaporated skim milk
   2. Fat: Homogenized milk, half-and-half

K. Soy or retextured protein

For Vegetarians

A. Very fat: All nuts and seeds

   Lean: Dried beans and peas, any soy protein or retextured protein

---

1. An ounce-for-ounce substitution (exchange) may be made once a day using lowfat yogurt for milk.

Vegetables

- asparagus[2]
- bean sprouts
- beets
- broccoli[2]
- brussels sprouts[2]
- cabbage
- carrots[2]
- cauliflower
- celery
- chard
- chicory
- Chinese cabbage
- collards[2]
- cucumbers
- dandelion greens[2]
- eggplant
- endive[2]
- escarole[2]
- green or red pepper
- kale[2]
- kohlrabi
- lettuce
- mushrooms
- mustard greens
- okra
- onions
- parsley
- radishes
- rhubarb
- rutabaga
- sauerkraut
- spinach[2]
- string beans
- summer squash
- tomatoes
- tomato juice
- turnips
- turnip greens[2]
- watercress
- winter squash[2] (butternut, acorn, etc.)

Fruits

- apple
- applesauce (unsweetened, ½ cup)
- apricots, fresh (2)
- banana (1 small)
- berries (½ cup)

---

2. These vegetables should be included in your menu at least 4-6 times a week.

cranberries (unsweetened)	orange juice (½ cup)
grapefruit	peach
grapefruit juice (½ cup)	pear
melon	persimmon
canteloupe (½ small)	pineapple (½ cup)
honeydew (¼ small)	pineapple juice (1/3 cup)
nectarine	pluns (2)
orange	tangerines

Grains (and grain substitutes)

Bread

Whole grain only: wheat, rye, soy, pumpernickel, etc.

Cereal

Bran, corn, rice, wheat germ, barley, wheat, shredded wheat

Grain Substitutes

Potato (1 small, approx. 3 oz.)

Winter Squash (acorn or butternut) may be used as a grain substitute only twice weekly, ½ cup.

Fats

Butter (and substitutes), 1 tsp. daily

Oil (safflower, peanut, corn, vegetable)

Salad dressing (with sugar listed fifth or below in ingredients)

Other

all sugar-free condiments	spices
diet soda	seasonings
fat-free bouillon	

FOOD LIST II

Proteins

Same as Food List I except:

Milk 8 oz. = ½ protein

Buttermilk 1 cup = ½ protein

Yogurt, lowfat, plain 1 cup = 1 protein

Vegetables (1 cup serving)

artichoke
asparagus
bean sprouts
broccoli
brussels sprouts
cabbage
cauliflower
celery
chard
cucumber
eggplant
greens (all types)
lettuce
mushrooms
okra
peppers (red, green)
radishes
parsley
pickles (not sweet)
sauerkraut
summer squash
tomatoes
turnips
zucchini

Limited Vegetables (½ cup)

beets
carrots
onions
pumpkin
rutabagas
winter squash
(acorn, buttermilk)

Grains

wheat germ (1/8 cup, substitute for 1 cup vegetable)

Fruit

- apple
- apricots (3 med.)
- blueberries (½ cup)
- boysenberries (1 cup)
- cantaloupe (½ small)
- casaba melon (¼ med.)
- cranberries (1 cup)
- grapefruit (½ med.)
- honeydew melon (¼ med.)
- lemons/limes (2)
- orange (1 med.)
- pineapple (½ cup)
- peach (1 med.)
- plums (2)
- raspberries (½ cup)
- strawberries (1 cup)
- tangerine (2 large)

Note: canned fruit may be eaten when fresh is not available, in half-cup portions.

Fats

- Butter (and substitutes), 1 tsp. daily
- Oil (safflower, peanut, corn, vegetable)
- Salad dressing (with sugar listed fifth or below in ingredients)

Other

- 3 tsp. lemon juice daily
- all sugar-free spices and condiments
- diet catsup and mustard

References and Resources

Benson, Herbert, M.D. *The Relaxation Response.* New York: William Morrow & Co., 1975.

Bray, George, M.D., ed. *Obesity in Perspective.* Bethesda, Md.: National Institutes of Health, 1973.

Build and Body Pressure Study. Chicago: Society of Actuaries, 1959.

Diagram Group, The. *The Complete Encyclopedia of Exercises.* New York & London: Paddington Press Ltd., 1979.

Dufty, William. *Sugar Blues.* New York: Warner Books, 1975.

Elliott, John. "Blame It All on Brown Fat Now," *Journal of the American Medical Association,* Vol. 243, pp. 1983–1985, 1980.

Food and Nutrition Board. *Recommended Dietary Allowances.* Washington: National Academy of Sciences, 1979.

Greenberg, Ira A. *Psychodrama: Theory and Therapy.* New York: Behavioral Publications, 1974.

Katz, Alfred H., and Bender, Eugene I. *The Strength in Us: Self-Help Groups in the Modern World.* New York: New Viewpoints, 1976.

Margules, David L.; Moisset, Beatriz; Lewis, Michael; Shibuya, Haruo; and Pert, Candace B. "B-Endorphin Is Associated with Overeating in Genetically Obese Mice (ob/ob) and Rats (fa/fa)," *Science,* Vol. 202, pp. 988–991, 1978.

Morehouse, Laurence E. and Gross, Leonard. *Total Fitness in Thirty Minutes a Week.* New York: Simon & Schuster, 1975.

Overeaters Anonymous. *A Program of Recovery,* Torrance, Calif.: Overeaters Anonymous, Inc., 1979.

Overeaters Anonymous. *Questions and Answers About Compulsive Overeating and the O.A. Program of Recovery.* Torrance, Calif.: Overeaters Anonymous, Inc., 1979.

Pipes, Thomas V., and Vodak, Paul A. *The Pipes Fitness Test & Prescription.* Los Angeles: J. P. Tarcher, Inc., 1978.

Royal Canadian Air Force Exercise Plans for Physical Fitness. New York: Pocket Books, 1972.

Shealy, C. Norman, M.D. *90 Days to Self-Health.* New York: Dial Press, 1977.

Smith, Manuel J. *When I Say No, I Feel Guilty.* New York: Dial Press, 1975.

Yablonsky, Lewis. *Psychodrama.* New York: Basic Books, 1976.

Index